Nouveau V

The New Renaissance of Vegan and Vegetarian Cuisine

Author

BEVERLY KUMARI

Contributing Authors

JJ LAYTON

ABDELLAH AGUENAOU

DOUGLAS DE LA REZA

ISBN 978-1-63575-861-0 (Hard Cover)
ISBN 978-1-63575-860-3 (Digital)

Copyright © 2017 by Beverly Kumari
All rights reserved. No part of this publication may be reproduced, distributed, or transmitted in any form or by any means, including photocopying, recording, or other electronic or mechanical methods without the prior written permission of the publisher. For permission requests, solicit the publisher via the address below.

Christian Faith Publishing, Inc.
296 Chestnut Street
Meadville, PA 16335
www.christianfaithpublishing.com

Printed in the United States of America

To my late husband, Newton H. Black; my late father, BJ, who reeled me into the wonderful world of culinary; and my mother, Betty, the original epicurean of our family.

—Beverly Kumari

To the three ladies in my life. May you always inspire me with passion and grace. Christy, Skylar, and Mom, I love you all.

—JJ Layton

To my dearest mother, who taught me all about food and service to others. Without you, none of this would be possible.

—Douglas De la Reza

Dedicated to my mother, wife, and children. Thank you for believing in me.

—Abdellah Aguenaou

Contents

Acknowledgments 3

Chapter 1   Salad Dressings and Marinades 5

Chapter 2   Sauces, Dips, and Stocks 21

Chapter 3   Appetizers 43

Chapter 4   Soups, Salads, and Sides 59

Chapter 5   Main Dishes 95

Chapter 6   Desserts 149

Chapter 7   Breakfast 163

Chapter 8   Breads 189

Index 199

About the Authors 204

ACKNOWLEDGMENTS

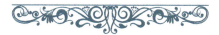

I thank the many people who assisted me in writing this cookbook. Executive Chef JJ Layton, who has been an avid supporter of this culinary journal and for mentoring me all along the way.

Executive Chef Doug De la Reza, for believing in my talent and allowing me to take the reins of my culinary career to a gastronomical level; one I thought was unreachable.

My father, BJ, who loved good food and gave me the tools, ambition, and drive I needed to live out loud.

My mother, Betty, who never seems to stop loving a new culinary challenge and instilling in me culinary etiquette.

My beautiful daughter, Erin, for whom I owe my entire life; you never stopped pushing me to shine.

And finally, my siblings, friends, and social media supporters, who incessantly motivate me to cook and write vegan and vegetarian recipes. Thank you for all being a part of this journey.

If I have failed to acknowledge anyone who has contributed to my writing this cookbook, please accept my apologies. I am forever grateful.

—Beverly Kumari

I would like to acknowledge all the culinarians, chefs, dish dogs, line warriors, and salad boys and girls for all your help and support; there are too many to mention. Thank you for allowing me to get where I am presently.

To my loving wife, family, and friends, thank you for the countless hours of support and trial runs of testing recipes that didn't always work out as planned. May your taste buds forgive me.

To Beverly, as iron sharpens iron, so have I grown assisting your culinary journey. It brings me great joy to be a part of this fantastic project.

—JJ Layton

To all those who have traversed with me throughout my culinary career, I am more than grateful for your avid support. Thank you, Beverly, for this great opportunity to work with you in creating a journal of bountiful recipes.

—Chef Douglas De la Reza

I acknowledge all those who have guided me along this path in assisting me in becoming an Executive Chef. I am forever grateful.

I would also like to thank the Culinary Institute of America and the Marriott for giving me one of the greatest opportunities in becoming the chef that I am today. Your guidance has allowed me to continually learn and develop new food concepts.

—Executive Chef Abdellah Aguenaou

CHAPTER 1

Salad Dressings and Marinades

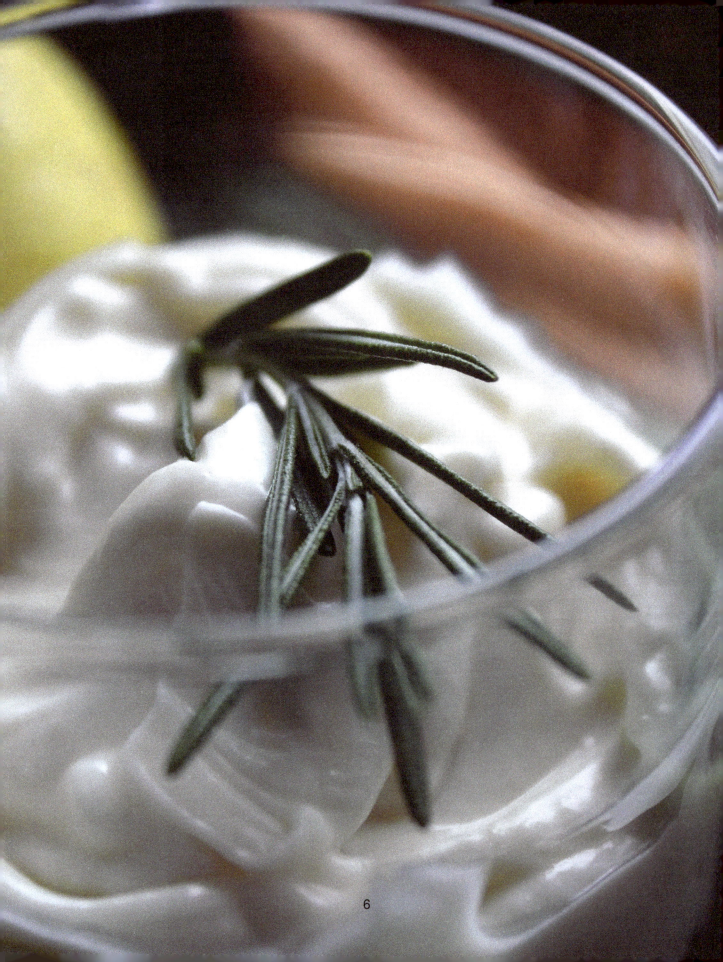

Veganaise

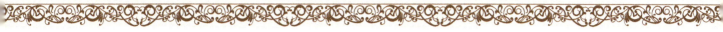

Ingredients:

- ½ cups full-fat soy milk (unsweetened and nonflavored)
- ¼ teaspoons apple cider vinegar
- ¼ teaspoons agave
- ¼ teaspoons lemon juice
- ¼ teaspoon Dijon mustard
- ½ cups grapeseed oil
- ½ cups plus 2 tablespoons extra-virgin olive oil
- Sea salt and black pepper to taste

Instructions:

Place all the ingredients except the oil in a blender and mix on high-speed until creamy and combined.

With your blender on a low speed, slowly stream in the oil to emulsify the mixture. Scrape down the sides of your blender, mix again, and season to taste, adding more salt, pepper, lemon, or mustard as needed.

If your mix comes out too thick, add a bit of almond milk. If it comes out too thin, add a bit more olive oil. It will thicken significantly as it chills in your fridge.

Varieties include the following: Add chopped cilantro; add 1 tablespoon wasabi powder; add ¼ cup minced roasted marinated red peppers; add 1 chopped chipotle pepper in adobo sauce; add 1 teaspoon of lime zest and 1 teaspoon of fresh lime juice; add 3 tablespoons of sriracha. You can always get creative and add your favorite ingredients, spices, and herbs.

Yields 2 to 3 servings

Buttermilk Yogurt Dressing

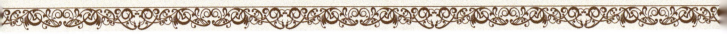

Ingredients:

½ cup buttermilk

2 ½ tablespoons Greek yogurt

½ teaspoon kosher salt

2 teaspoons freshly squeezed lemon juice

2 teaspoons agave

fresh ground pepper to taste

Instructions:

Combine the buttermilk, yogurt and, salt, lemon juice, and agave. Whisk together, making sure all ingredients are incorporated. Add pepper, and refrigerate until use.

Yields 2 to 3 servings

Basic Vinaigrette

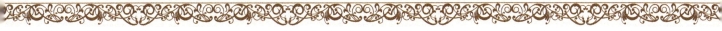

Ingredients:

- ¾ cup olive oil
- 3–4 tablespoons fresh lemon juice
- 1 ¼ teaspoon Dijon mustard
- ½ teaspoon kosher salt
- ¼ teaspoon white pepper

Instructions:

In a stainless steel mixing bowl, whisk together lemon juice, Dijon mustard, salt, and white pepper until all ingredients are incorporated.

Stream the olive oil into the mixed ingredients until the vinaigrette becomes emulsified (thickened).

Yields 2 to 3 servings

Balsamic Vinaigrette

Ingredients:

¾ cup olive oil
3 tablespoons balsamic
1 tablespoon of honey
1 garlic clove, minced
1 ¼ teaspoon Dijon mustard
½ teaspoon kosher salt
¼ teaspoon white pepper

Instructions:

In a stainless steel mixing bowl, whisk together balsamic, honey, Dijon mustard, minced garlic, salt, and white pepper until all ingredients are incorporated.

Stream the olive oil into the mixed ingredients until the vinaigrette becomes emulsified (thickened).

Yields 2 to 3 servings

Champagne Vinaigrette

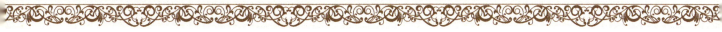

Ingredients:

- 1 garlic clove, finely chopped
- 2 tablespoons Dijon mustard
- ¼ cup white balsamic vinegar
- ½ cup champagne or white sparkling wine
- 2 tablespoons honey
- ½ teaspoon salt
- ½ teaspoon freshly ground black pepper
- ½ cup extra virgin olive oil

Instructions:

In a stainless steel bowl, whisk together the garlic, mustard, vinegar, champagne, honey, salt, and pepper.

Stream in olive oil, and slowly whisk until the dressing is emulsified.

Yields 2 to 3 servings

Dijon Vinaigrette

Ingredients:

1 tablespoon fresh lemon juice
1 teaspoon Dijon mustard
1 tablespoon white balsamic vinegar
1 garlic clove, finely minced
½ cup extra virgin olive oil
sea salt and white pepper to taste
freshly ground black pepper

Instructions:

In a stainless steel bowl, whisk lemon juice, Dijon mustard, vinegar, and garlic in a medium bowl.

Stream in the olive oil, and whisk until the vinaigrette is emulsified. Season to taste with salt and pepper.

Yields 2 to 3 servings

Herb Oil Marinade

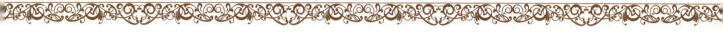

Ingredients:

- 2 medium shallots, peeled and roughly chopped
- 5 garlic cloves, peeled and smashed
- 1 bunch parsley, roughly chopped
- 1 bunch oregano, roughly chopped
- 15 sprigs of rosemary, destemmed
- 15 sprigs of thyme, destemmed
- 2 ½ cups extra virgin olive oil

Instructions:

In a blender or food processor, pulse the shallot, garlic, and herbs to combine. Add the olive oil, then pulse until a smooth sauce forms.

Transfer the sauce to an airtight container, and refrigerate until ready to use.

Yields 18 ounces

Barbecue Sauce

Ingredients:

2 cups ketchup

¼ cup dark brown sugar

1 teaspoon granulated garlic

1 teaspoon onion powder

juice of freshly squeezed lemon juice

1 tablespoon of tamari

1 tablespoon smoked paprika

2 dashes of liquid smoke

2 dashes of sriracha

salt and pepper to taste

Instructions:

Combine all ingredients in a saucepan, and heat over medium-high heat, stirring to mix all ingredients well. Turn down heat to medium, and let sauce simmer for about 10 to 12 minutes. Serve with vegetables, or your favorite veggie meatless products.

Yields 18 ounces

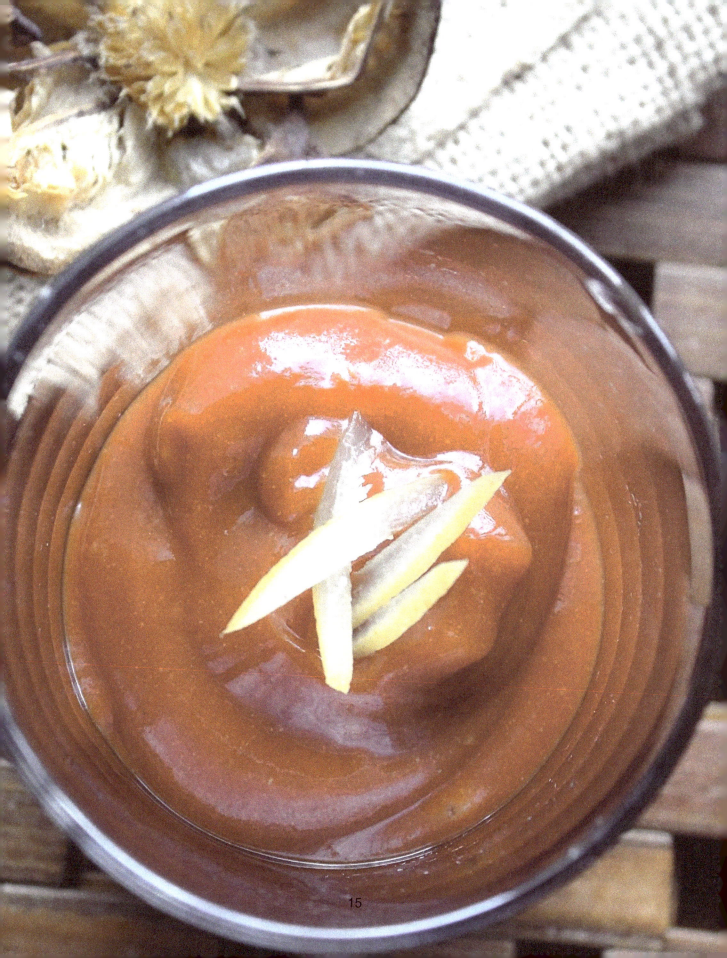

Tamari Ginger Marinade

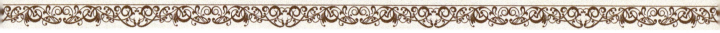

Ingredients:

- ½ tablespoons tamari sauce
- 1 teaspoon onion powder
- 1 teaspoon granulated garlic
- 1 tablespoon minced ginger
- 1 tablespoon sesame seed oil
- 1 tablespoon of agave
- 1 teaspoon red pepper flakes

Instructions:

In a bowl, mix together all ingredients until well combined. Cover, and refrigerate until further use.

Use as a marinade with tofu, vegetables, or your favorite meatless products.

Yields 2 to 3 servings

Chermoula

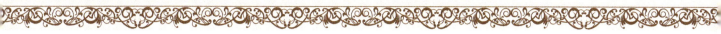

Ingredients:

½ cup (or to taste) fresh lemon juice (or ¼ cup lemon juice and ¼ cup wine vinegar)
6 cloves garlic, very finely minced
2 teaspoons sweet paprika or pimenton dulce
½ teaspoon cayenne pepper
2 teaspoons ground toasted cumin
¼ cup chopped fresh parsley
¼ cup chopped cilantro
1 cup extra virgin olive oil, or as needed
Salt and freshly ground pepper
Optional: chopped preserved lemon

Instructions:

To make chermoula, mix the lemon juice, garlic, paprika, cayenne, and cumin in a mixing bowl until smooth. Whisk in the parsley, cilantro, and olive oil.

To make chermoula vinaigrette, mix the lemon juice, garlic, paprika, cayenne, and cumin in a mixing bowl until smooth. Whisk in the parsley, cilantro, and olive oil. If necessary, add more oil so that the vinaigrette is not too thick. Taste and add more lemon juice or vinegar if needed.

Season with salt and pepper.

Yields 2 to 3 servings

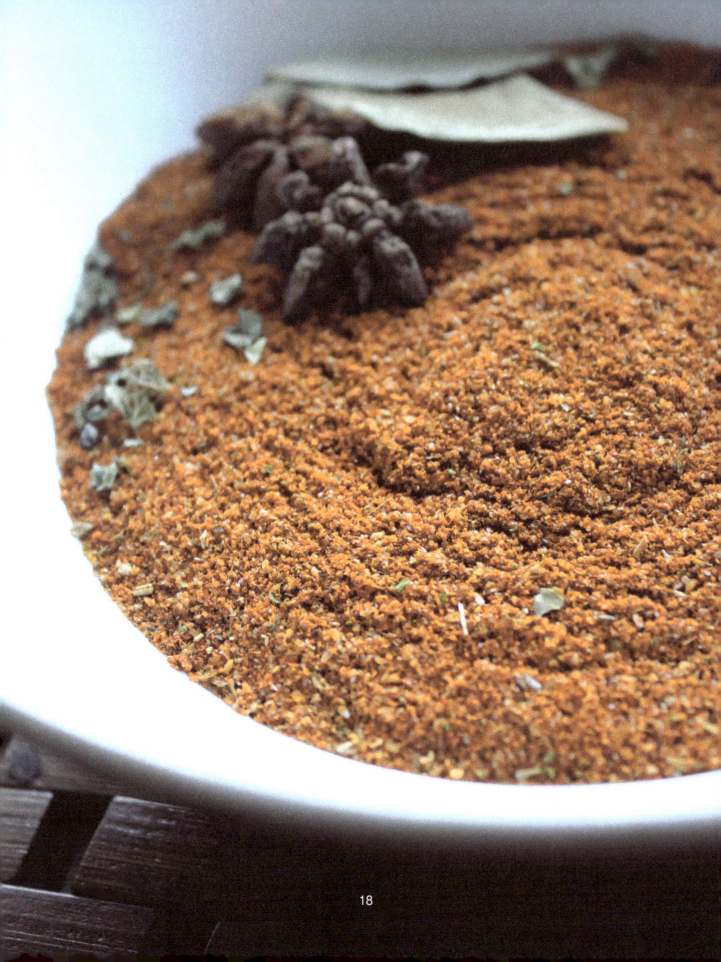

Moroccan Spice Mix

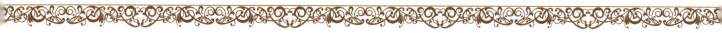

Ingredients:

- paprika powder, 3 ounces
- cumin powder, 2 ounces
- coriander powder, 1 ounce
- chili powder, 1 ounce
- cayenne powder, 1 teaspoon

Instructions:

If using seeds, blend all ingredients in a coffee grinder, and mix all together. Otherwise, if using powdered ingredients, combine all and mix well. Seal in an airtight container for later usage.

Yields approximately 8 ounces

CHAPTER 2

Sauces, Dips, and Stocks

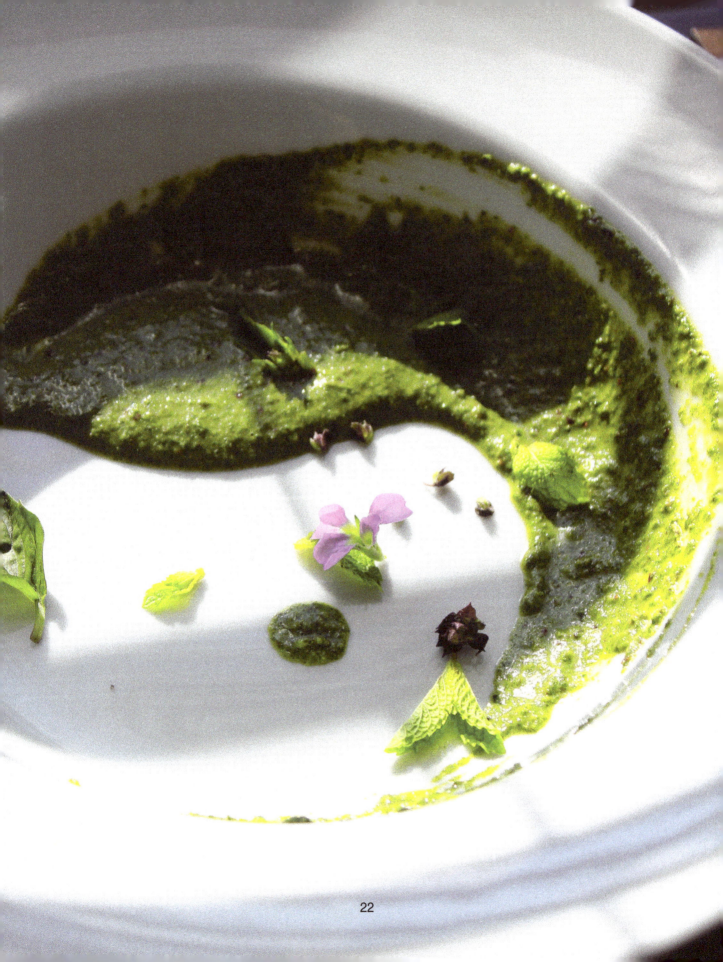

Chef Bev's Chimichurri

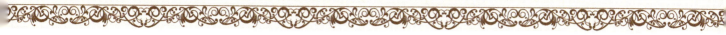

Ingredients:

1 cup lightly packed fresh mint
1 cup lightly packed fresh basil (I prefer Thai basil as it is more aromatic)
½ cup lightly packed fresh oregano
¼ teaspoon crushed red pepper flakes
1 teaspoon honey (light agave if you are vegan)
4 garlic cloves
2 tablespoons red wine vinegar
1 ½ cups of extra virgin olive oil
salt and pepper to taste

Instructions:

In a food processor, combine honey, red pepper flakes, red wine vinegar, mint, basil, oregano, and garlic. Process until finely chopped.

With motor running, gradually pour oil through the feed tube. Season with salt and pepper. Serve with your favorite veggies, breads, or vegan proteins.

Yields 18 ounces

Tomato Glaze

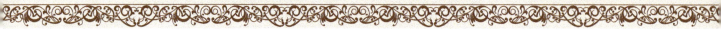

Ingredients:

- 4 teaspoons olive oil
- ¼ cups tomato paste
- 1 cup tomato sauce
- 2 tablespoons cider vinegar
- 2 teaspoons agave or honey
- 2 teaspoons Worcestershire sauce
- 1 tablespoon Dijon mustard
- 1 tablespoon balsamic vinegar
- ¼ teaspoons table salt
- ¼ teaspoons table white pepper

Instructions:

Heat olive oil in pot on stove stop over medium heat. Add remaining ingredients, and whisk over medium heat until the mixture is smooth and without lumps. Serve with your favorite meatless loaf or chickenless or porkless dish.

Yields approximately 1 ¾ cups

Mojo Sauce

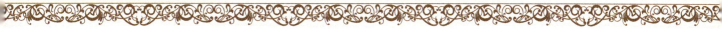

Ingredients:

- 2 garlic cloves, peeled
- 2 teaspoons paprika
- 1 teaspoon cumin
- 5 tablespoons extra virgin olive oil
- 2 tablespoons white wine vinegar

Instructions:

Add garlic, paprika, cumin, and white wine vinegar to the bowl of a food processor, and process until the mixture is smooth.

Gradually add the extra virgin olive oil through the feeder tube until it is well blended and slightly emulsified.

Yields approximately ½ cups

Blond Vegetable Stock

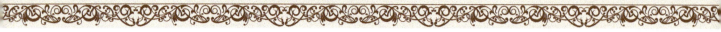

Ingredients:

- 3 onions, roughly chopped
- 3 stalk celery, roughly chopped
- 2 carrots, roughly chopped
- 1 bay leaf
- 10 peppercorns, whole
- ¼ cups kosher sea salt
- 1 sheet kombu or nori
- 1 garlic clove
- 1 tablespoon coconut oil
- 2 ½ quarts filtered water

Instructions:

Heat a large stock pot over medium-high heat. Add coconut oil. When oil begins to simmer, add onions, celery, and carrot. Stir to caramelize on all sides, for approximately 10 minutes.

Add remaining ingredients. Cover and allow stock to come to a boil. Reduce to medium low, and simmer stock for 45 minutes.

Pass stock through chinois, and reserve vegetables for another use.

Yields approximately 2 quarts

Brown Vegetable Stock

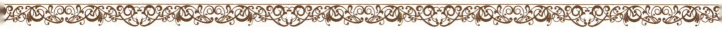

Ingredients:

3 onions, roughly chopped

3 celery stalks, roughly chopped

2 carrots, roughly chopped

4 garlic cloves

1 tablespoon coconut oil

¼ cup dried mushroom powder

1 bay leaf

10 peppercorns, whole

¼ cup kosher sea salt

1 sheet kombu or nori

2 ½ quarts filtered water

Instructions:

Combine onions, celery, carrots, and garlic in a mixing bowl.

Coat with coconut oil, and place on a cooking sheet.

Roast in a 315-degree convection oven for 90 minutes. (If using a conventional/household oven, increase cooking time to 2 ½ hours.)

Add to a stockpot with remaining ingredients, and bring to a slow boil. Simmer for 45 minutes.

Pass through a chinois, and discard vegetable pulp. (Pass through a coffee filter if an extremely fine stock is desired.)

Yields approximately 2 quarts

White Wine Sauce

Ingredients:

- 3 shallots, finely minced
- ¼ cups white wine
- 1 tablespoon of white wine vinegar
- 4 tablespoons butter
- pinch of salt to taste
- ½ teaspoons freshly chopped parsley

Instructions:

In a small saucepan, sauté shallot in 1 tablespoon of olive oil until translucent. Continue cooking over low heat, stirring occasionally. Add wine and reduce. Continue to cook for about 15 minutes.

Allow to cool. Stir in parsley.

Whisk in some room-temperature butter, stirring over low heat. Add salt, vinegar.

Yields approximately ½ cups

Chef Bev's Romesco Sauce

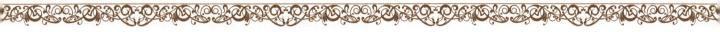

Ingredients:

1 large marinated roasted red bell pepper

1 tablespoon of garlic paste

½ cups toasted slivered almonds

¼ cups tomato paste

2 tablespoons chopped parsley

2 tablespoons of chopped oregano

½ cup grated parmesan cheese

2 tablespoons sherry vinegar

1 teaspoon smoked paprika

½ teaspoons cayenne pepper

½ cups extra virgin olive oil

sea salt and freshly ground black pepper

Instructions:

Pulse first 10 ingredients in a food processor until very finely chopped. With motor running, slowly add oil; process until smooth. Season with salt and pepper.

Yields 2 to 3 servings

Alfredo Sauce

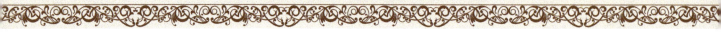

Ingredients:

¼ pound unsalted butter

1 tablespoon extra virgin olive oil

½ cup of dry white wine

1 tablespoon Italian herbs

1 medium-sized shallot small dice

1 tablespoon garlic paste

1 cup heavy cream

¾ cup parmesan cheese, freshly grated

salt and pepper to taste

¼ teaspoon nutmeg

Instructions:

Heat butter and oil in pan until melted. Add shallots and garlic paste, and stir for about 5 minutes until shallots are translucent. Add wine, and reduce by 50%, or until half of the wine has evaporated.

Add cream after the wine has been reduced to half, and then stir in parmesan cheese (making sure to constantly stir the mixture so the cream won't scorch and cheese will not burn). Stir until the cheese has melted.

Add salt and pepper to taste as well as the nutmeg.

Serve immediately.

Yields 2 to 3 servings

Cucumber Cilantro Sauce

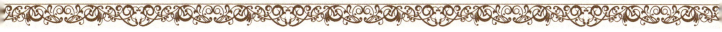

Ingredients:

    1 cup fresh cilantro, chopped
    1 cup diced, peeled cucumber
    ½ cup lemon juice
    ¼ cup olive oil
    ½ teaspoon salt

Instructions:

Puree the cilantro, cucumber, lemon juice, olive oil, and salt in the food processor or blender until smooth with just a bit of texture.

Yields 2 to 3 servings

Tomato Sauce

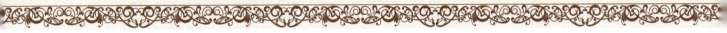

Ingredients:

- 2 cups onions, diced
- 1 cup carrots, diced
- 1 cup celery, diced
- 1 clove garlic, minced
- 2 28-ounce cans crushed tomatoes
- 1 quart vegetable stock
- kosher salt, to taste
- sugar, to taste

Instructions:

Heat olive oil in pot on stove stop over medium heat. Add remaining ingredients, and whisk over medium heat until the mixture is smooth and without lumps. Serve with your favorite meatless loaf or chickenless or porkless dish.

Yields approximately 2 quarts

Lemon Dill Sauce

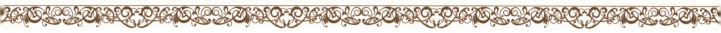

Ingredients:

½ cup minced shallots

1 teaspoon minced garlic

½ cup dry white wine

juice of one lemon

¼ cups chopped fresh dill

1 teaspoon Dijon mustard

½ cups heavy cream

5 tablespoons unsalted butter, cubed

salt and pepper

Instructions:

In a saucepan, combine the shallots, garlic, wine, and lemon. Bring the liquid up to a boil. Stir in the dill, and cook for 3 minutes. Whisk in the mustard and cream; continue to cook for 2 minutes. Whisk in the butter a cube at a time, until all the butter is incorporated. Season with salt and pepper.

Yields 2 to 3 servings

Sun-Dried Tomato and Roasted Garlic Sauce

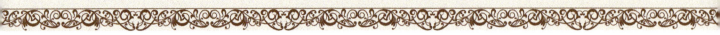

Ingredients:

- 5 medium-to-large roasted garlic cloves (peeled)
- 3 tablespoons of extra virgin olive oil
- ½ cups julienned sun dried tomatoes
- 1 ½ cups tomato passata
- ½ teaspoons of sea salt (kosher preferably)
- 1 ½ tablespoons raw sugar
- 1 teaspoon fresh oregano

Instructions:

Roast garlic in 350-degree oven for about 20 minutes.

Heat oil in Dutch oven over medium heat, and add peeled roasted garlic and sun-dried tomatoes, stirring to make sure garlic does not stick to the bottom of the pot.

Add the tomato sauce, and stir to incorporate ingredients, again stirring to make sure there is no scorching or sticking of the sauce and ingredients.

Add sea salt, raw sugar, and oregano. Stir the ingredients together. Turn heat down to a low simmer. Cook for about 45 minutes.

Yields 2 to 3 servings

Roasted Eggplant with Gorgonzola Cheese Pasta Sauce

Ingredients:

2 medium minced garlic cloves

¼ cups minced onion1 teaspoon extra virgin olive oil

⅓ cups julienned and roasted eggplant

½ teaspoons of salt (kosher, preferably)

pinch of white pepper

¼ cups heavy cream

1 chopped basil leaf

¼ cups of gorgonzola cheese (crumbled)

Instructions:

Roast medium julienned eggplant in a sauté pan with the olive oil until nice and gold.

Add minced garlic and minced onion, stirring frequently, making sure garlic does not burn and the onions caramelize. Add salt and a pinch of white pepper.

Add the heavy cream, salt, and chopped basil. Stir the ingredients together, and then add the gorgonzola cheese, stirring frequently.

Turn heat down to a low simmer. Cook for about 45 minutes, or until all the ingredients are emulsified and incorporated.

Yields 2 to 3 servings

Grilled Artichoke Marinara Parmigiano

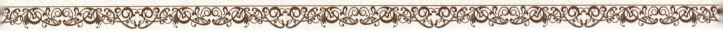

Ingredients:

- 2 medium minced garlic cloves
- 2 tablespoons of extra virgin olive oil
- ½ cups grilled and quartered artichoke hearts
- ½ teaspoons of sea salt (kosher, preferably)
- ½ tablespoons raw sugar
- pinch of white pepper
- 1 ½ cups passata sauce
- 1 teaspoon chopped rosemary leaf
- ¼ cups of 24-month-aged grated parmesan cheese

Instructions:

Grill artichoke hearts whole, turning frequently so as not burn. I usually use an indoor grill (George Foreman) as it is smokeless and easy to clean.

Heat the oil in Dutch oven over medium heat, and add minced garlic, stirring frequently, making sure garlic does not burn. Add salt and a pinch of black pepper.

Add grilled artichokes, and then add the tomato sauce, sea salt, raw sugar, and chopped rosemary. Stir the ingredients together, and then add the grated parmesan cheese.

Turn heat down to a low simmer. Cook for about 45 minutes.

Yields 2 to 3 servings

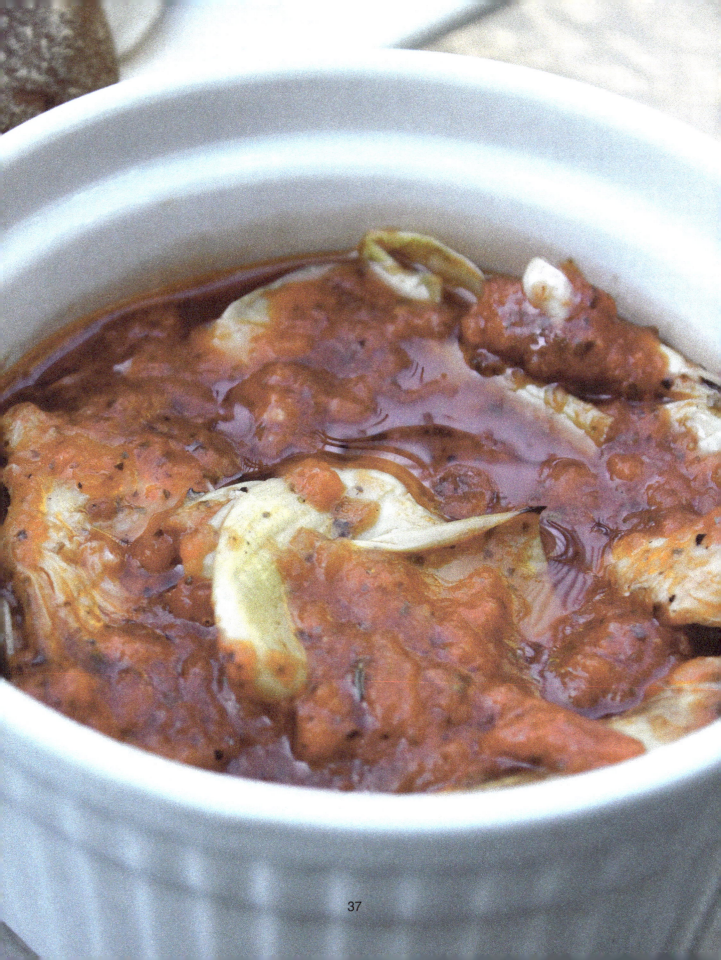

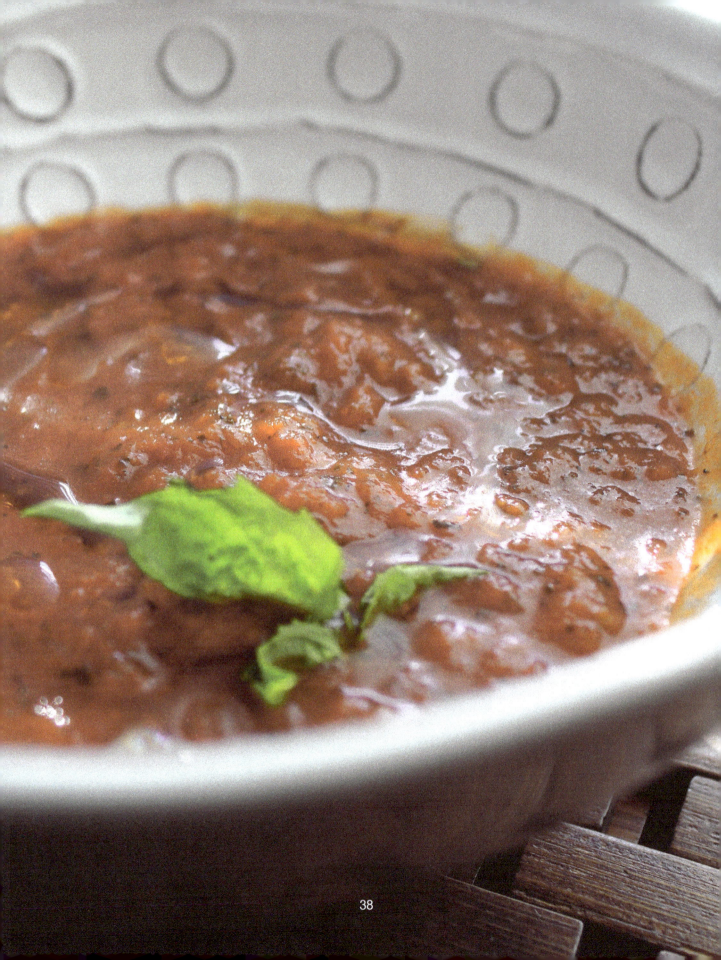

Classic Marinara Sauce

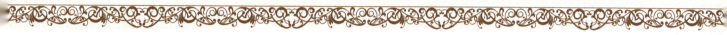

Ingredients:

- 2 medium minced garlic cloves
- 2 tablespoons of extra virgin olive oil
- ½ teaspoons of sea salt (kosher, preferably)
- ¼ tablespoons raw sugar
- 1 ½ cups classic tomato sauce
- ¼ cups red wine (cabernet sauvignon)
- 1 chopped basil leaf
- ¼ cups of 24-month-aged grated parmesan cheese

Instructions:

Heat the oil in Dutch oven over medium heat, and add minced garlic, stirring frequently, making sure garlic does not burn. Add tomato sauce, red wine, sea salt, raw sugar, and chopped basil. Stir the ingredients together, and then add the grated parmesan cheese.

Turn heat down to a low simmer. Cook for about 45 minutes.

Yields 2 to 3 servings

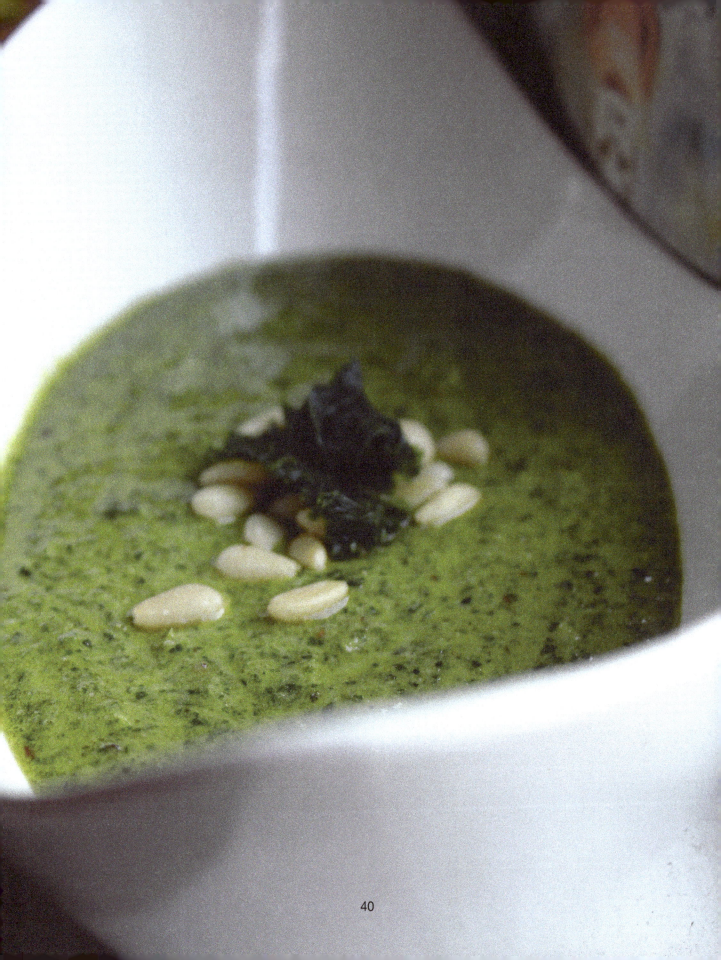

Kale and Tarragon Pesto

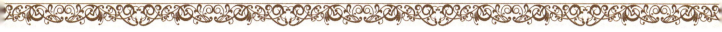

Ingredients:

1 ½ cups kale, destemmed and roughly chopped

½ bunch tarragon, destemmed

½ cup walnuts, chopped

½ cup nutritional yeast

2 garlic cloves

juice from 1 large lemon, plus ¼ teaspoon of lemon zest

¼ cup extra virgin olive oil

1 teaspoon of salt to cook kale

salt and pepper to taste

Instructions:

In a large pot, bring 3 cups of water to a rapid boil, and add 1 teaspoon of salt. Add the kale, and cook for 7 minutes. Remove from heat, and drain the kale. Let cool for about 10 minutes.

In a food processor or blender, combine the kale, tarragon, walnuts, garlic nutritional yeast, olive oil, and lemon juice. Process until smooth. Add salt and pepper and more lemon to taste.

Yields 2 to 3 servings

Chapter 3

Appetizers

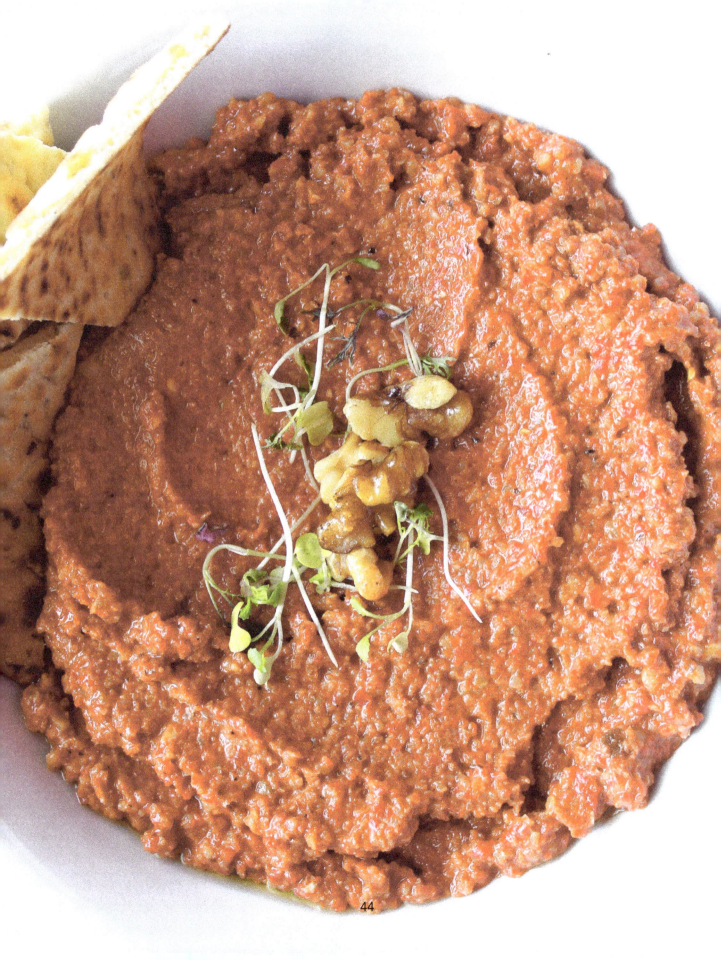

Muhammara

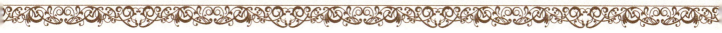

Ingredients:

- 2 red bell peppers
- 1 cup walnuts, toasted
- 1 clove garlic, roughly chopped
- juice of ½ lemon
- ¼ cup bread crumbs
- 1 tablespoon pomegranate molasses
- 1 teaspoon smoked paprika
- ½ teaspoon red pepper flakes
- ¼ teaspoon cumin
- 2 tablespoons olive oil

Instructions:

Preheat oven broiler.

Cut peppers in half, and remove stems and seeds. Line a baking sheet with parchment paper, and place peppers on it, skin side up. Broil peppers until skins are charred, approximately 12 to 15 minutes. Remove from oven, and using a pair of tongs, place the peppers in a paper bag. Seal and set aside until peppers are cool enough to handle, about 10–15 minutes.

Once peppers have cooled, peel off and discard most of the charred black skins.

Add the roasted peeled pepper halves to the bowl of a food processor, along with remaining ingredients, with the exception of the olive oil. Blend to combine.

Stream the olive oil into the mixture from the opening of the food processor bowl. I like my muhammara a bit chunky, so I only pulse a few times to give it the texture it needs to be chunky. However, you may blend the mixture to your desired consistency.

Scrape into a serving bowl, and serve with warm pita bread.

Yields 2 to 3 servings

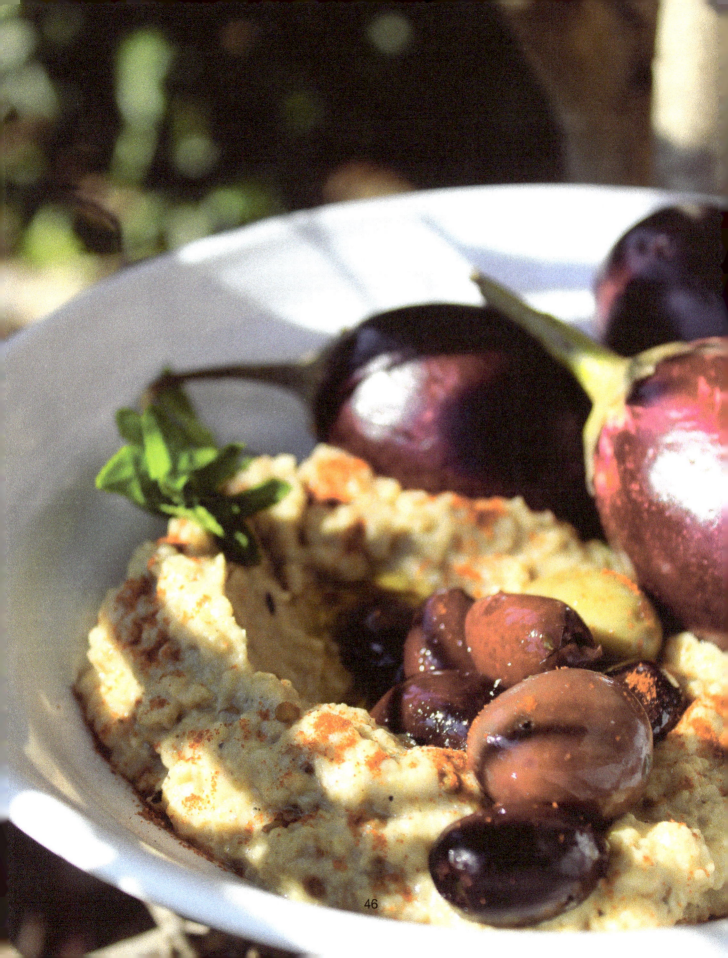

Baba Ghanouj

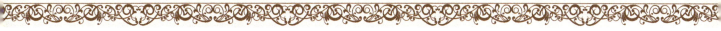

Ingredients:

- 3–5 medium eggplants (3 pounds)
- 5 tablespoons tahini paste
- juice from 1 freshly squeezed lemon
- 3 garlic cloves, crushed
- 1 table spoon white vinegar
- 1 teaspoon salt or to taste
- 1 tablespoon extra virgin olive oil
- pinch of cumin
- chopped parsley for garnish
- paprika for garnish-

Instructions:

Puncture the skins of the eggplants with a fork, and roast in a 400 degree oven for 35 to 40 minutes.

While eggplants are still hot, peel them, and discard the seeds.

Strain the water from the eggplants by placing them in a colander for about 10 minutes. This step is important so you don't get a liquid baba ghanouj.

Add eggplants and all ingredients to the bowl of a food processor, and let run for 2–3 minutes until you get a paste.

Place baba ghanouj paste into a serving plate. Garnish extra virgin oil, chopped parsley, and paprika.

Serve with pita bread.

Yields 2 to 3 servings

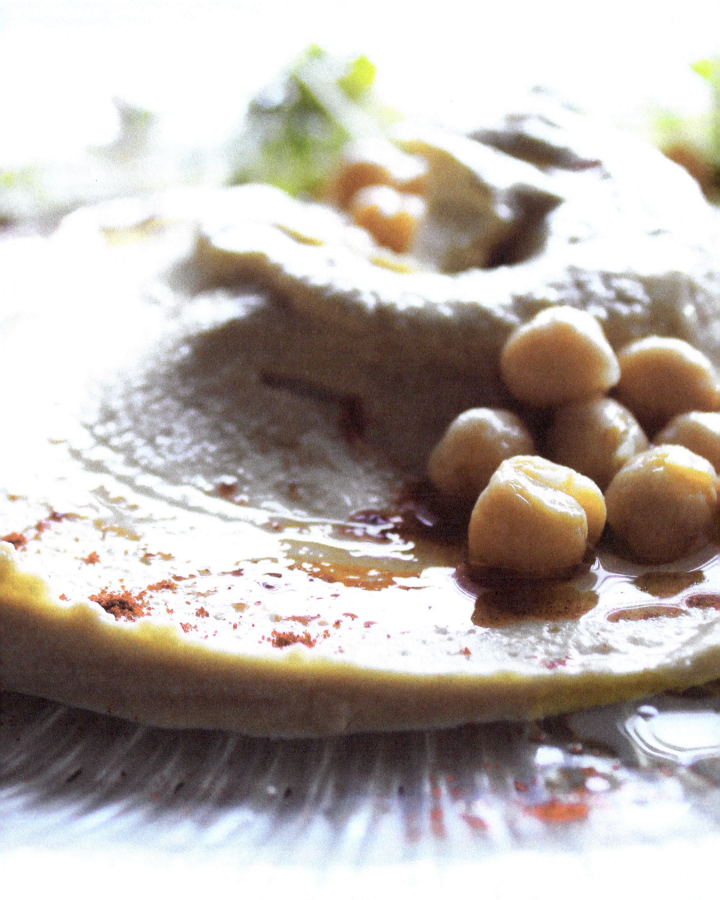

Hummus

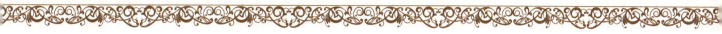

Ingredients:

1 16-ounce can of chickpeas, drained and rinsed well

4 tablespoons tahini paste

juice of one freshly squeezed lemon

2 garlic cloves

½ tsp salt

pinch of cumin

2 tablespoons plain Greek yogurt or plain unflavored vegan yogurt

dash of paprika for garnish

saffron-infused extra virgin olive oil for drizzling

Instructions:

Drain, wash chickpeas, and place them in a medium-size pot. Cover and cook for 17 to 20 minutes until the chickpeas are soft. Once fully cooked, transfer chickpeas immediately to a large sieve or colander over your sink. Run cold water as you rub chickpeas by the handful to remove the skin.

Place tahini, lemon juice, and garlic cloves in a food processor. Pulse for a few seconds to combine. Now add the cooked chickpeas, cumin, salt, and Greek yogurt (or vegan yogurt). Puree until you achieve a smooth and creamy hummus dip.

Serve at room temperature, or cooler, topped with saffron-infused olive oil and a dash of paprika. Serve with pita bread or a crudité of vegetables.

Yields 2 to 3 servings

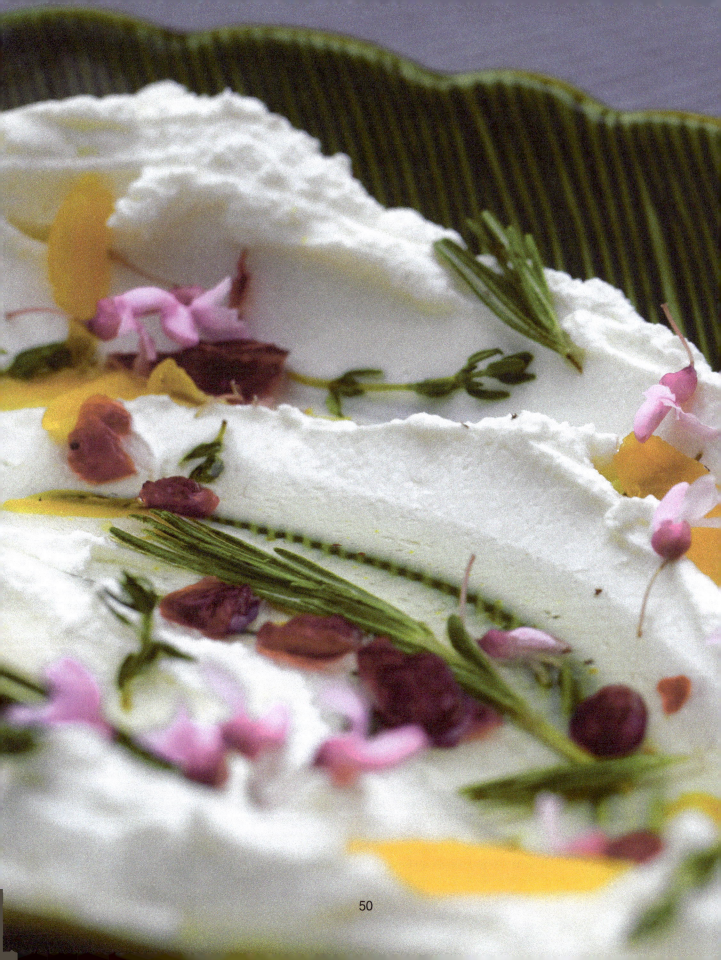

Chef Bev's Labneh

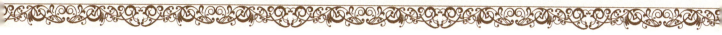

Ingredients:

32 ounces of Greek yogurt

juice of 1 freshly squeezed lemon

1 teaspoon kosher salt

pinch of white pepper

extra virgin olive oil

¼ cup sliced julienned dried apricots

fresh herbs, and edible flowers for garnish

Instructions:

Place a piece of doubled cheesecloth in the bottom of a colander, and then place the colander over a deep bowl.

Stir the salt, white pepper, and lemon juice into the yogurt. Place the combined ingredients and yogurt into the center of the cheesecloth.

Leave to drain for 4 to 5 hours. When the labneh is well drained, it should be the consistency of cream cheese.

Garnish the labneh with extra virgin olive oil and fresh herbs. Serve with a crusty warm boule of bread.

Yields 2 to 3 servings

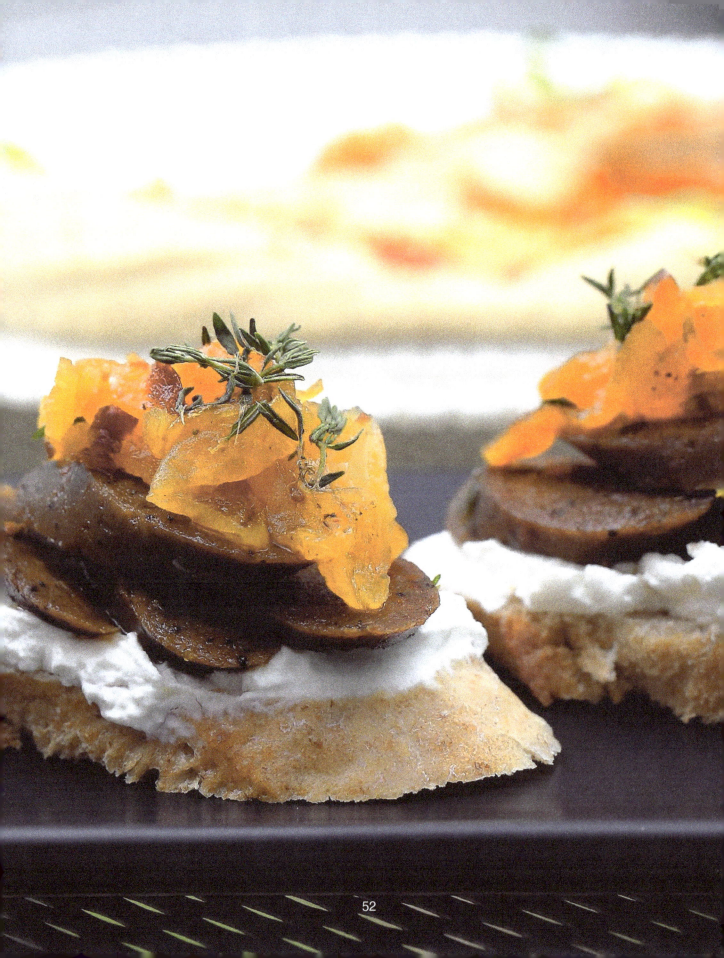

Labneh Crostini with Tofurkey Italian Sausage, Dried Apricots, and Thyme

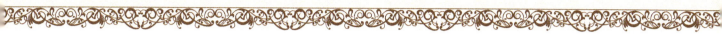

Ingredients:

- 4 Tofurkey Italian sausage links, sliced on the bias
- ¼ cup dried apricots, julienned
- 3 sprigs of thyme
- ¾ cups labneh (recipe on page 51)
- 1 mini French baguette, cut on the bias into 12 slices
- 2 tablespoons of extra virgin olive oil plus 2 tablespoons more

Instructions:

Heat a sauté pan over medium-high heat, and add 2 tablespoons of extra virgin olive oil. Add Tofurkey Italian sausage, julienned apricots, and thyme. Sauté for about 5 to 7 minutes until the Tofurkey is browned and the apricots are soft and slightly caramelized. Remove Tofurkey, sauté from heat, and set aside.

Preheat oven to 375 degrees.

Place baguette slices on a nonstick sheet pan, and place into the oven for 2 to 3 minutes. Remove from oven, and set aside to cool for 5 to 10 minutes.

Spread 1 tablespoon each on the baguette slices. Spoon on the Tofurkey, apricot, and thyme mixture onto each labneh and baguette slice.

Drizzle the remaining extra virgin olive oil onto each crostini. Garnish with any additional sprigs of thyme.

Yields 4 to 6 servings

Sicilian Caponata

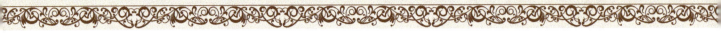

Ingredients:

- 5 eggplants cut into bite-size cubes
- 15 green olives, pitted and halved
- 2 tablespoons capers, rinsed
- 3 tablespoons extra virgin olive oil
- 2 large onions, chopped
- 1 16-ounce box of pomi chopped tomatoes with liquid
- 3 celery stalks, chopped
- ¼ cup chopped basil
- 150 ml, or up to 5 ounces red wine vinegar
- 1 tablespoon brown sugar
- ½ tablespoons balsamic vinegar
- ¼ cup golden raisins

Instructions:

Pour hot water over raisins in a small bowl, and set aside to plump while you do your prep work. Heat a large skillet over medium heat, and add 2 tablespoons of olive oil. When the oil has become hot, add eggplant cubes and arrange in a single layer as much as possible. Cook for about 10 minutes, gently turning occasionally until the eggplant is browned on all sides.

Transfer to a bowl with a slotted spoon.

Reduce heat to medium, and add the remaining 1 tablespoon of oil to the pan. Saute the onions, and celery for about 3 minutes, stirring frequently to avoid burning. Add garlic, and cook for approximately 1 minute.

Add tomato and cook for about 2 minutes, stirring frequently. Gently fold eggplant back into the pan with the tomato mixture, along with red wine vinegar, raisins, sugar, balsamic, capers, and olives.

Remove from heat, and season with salt and pepper. Add basil, and gently stir to combine. Serve warm or at room temperature. Caponata will keep in a sealed container in the refrigerator for a few days. Bring to room temperature before serving.

Yields 4 to 6 servings

Mini Black Bean Cakes

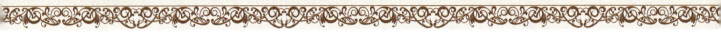

Ingredients:

- 2 ½ tablespoons of chickpea flour
- 2 15-ounce cans black beans, drained and rinsed
- 2 medium garlic cloves, finely chopped
- ¼ cup coconut milk
- ½ cups fine, unseasoned panko
- ½ cups coarsely chopped fresh cilantro
- ½ cups small-diced white onion
- 1 tablespoon plus 1 teaspoon sriracha
- ½ lime, zested on microplane
- 1 teaspoon kosher sea salt
- 1 teaspoon black pepper, fresh ground
- ½ cups blended oil

Instructions:

Place the beans, garlic, coconut milk, bread crumbs, cilantro, onion, hot sauce, and salt in a food processor fitted with a blade attachment. Pulse until the ingredients are incorporated and the beans are broken down but some whole beans remain, about 15 (1-second) pulses, stopping the processor and scraping down the sides of the bowl with a rubber spatula as needed. Add the chickpea flour to the mixture, and mix well.

Scoop the bean mixture into your hands 1 heaping tablespoon at a time, and form it into 24 (2-inch-wide) patties.

Heat ¼ cups of the oil in a large frying pan over medium-high heat until shimmering, about 4 minutes. Place 8 of the patties in the pan, and fry until golden brown and heated through, adjusting the heat as necessary, about 3 minutes per side.

Return the fried patties to the baking sheet, and repeat with the remaining patties, adding the remaining oil to the pan as needed between batches. Place the baking sheet in the oven to keep warm.

Garnish with lime zest.

Yields 6 to 8 servings

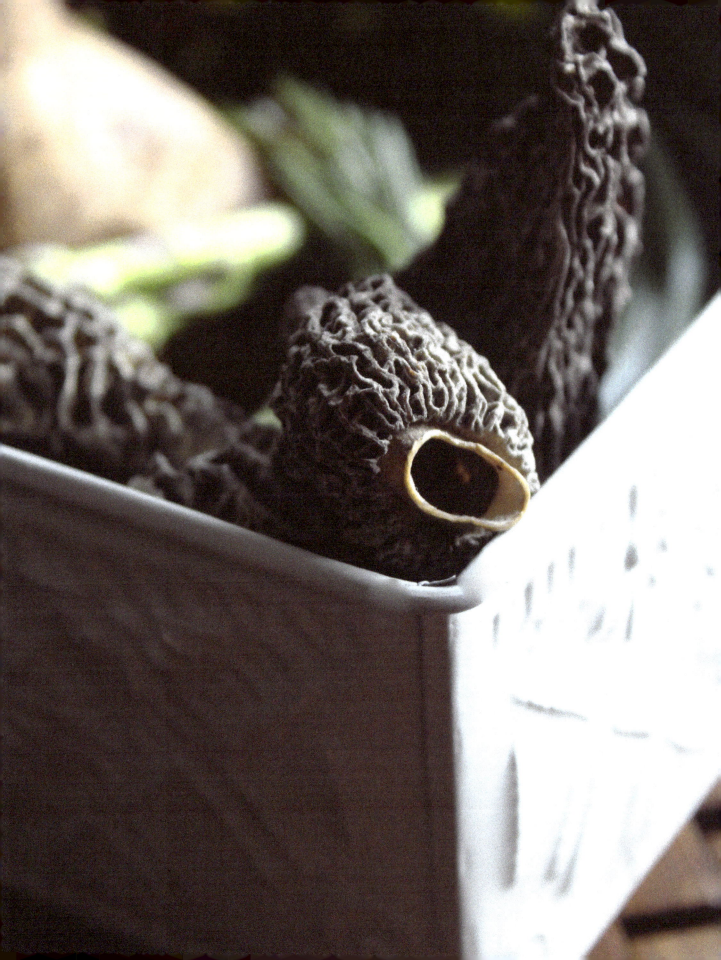

Chapter 4

Soups, Salads, and Sides

Papaya Gazpacho

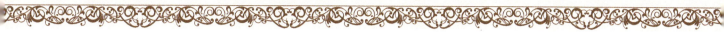

Ingredients:

5 cups peeled, seeded and roughly chopped papaya, plus 1 cup medium dice
½ cups papaya nectar
1 teaspoon agave
1 tablespoon of white balsamic vinegar
1 cup peeled, seeded, and diced cucumber
1 cup diced celery (about 2 stalks)
¾ cup diced red bell pepper (about 1 pepper)
1 teaspoon jalapenos, small dice
¼ cups fresh mint leaves, minced
¼ cups fresh cilantro, minced
juice of 1 lemon (about 3 tablespoons)
salt and white pepper to taste

Orange Papaya Foam

½ cup cold orange juice
½ cup cold papaya nectar

Instructions:

Combine 5 cups papaya and the papaya nectar into a food processor or blender, and puree until mixture is smooth but slightly chunky. You should have 3 ½ cups strained liquid and pulp.

Add cucumber, celery, bell pepper, minced mint and cilantro, lemon juice, vinegar, agave, jalapeno, and remaining cup of diced papaya to strained papaya and orange juice mixture. Stir to combine. Refrigerate for 1 hour or more so that the flavors meld.

To make the orange papaya foam, place cold orange juice and cold papaya nectar in a stainless steel mixing bowl. Using an immersion blender, blend the juice mixture, beginning at the bottom on high speed for about 2 minutes. Gradually bring the blender just before the top of the juice mixture, skimming the top to create a foam. Blend on high speed for an additional 3 to 5 minutes until the foam has doubled in size.

To serve gazpacho, ladle the chilled soup into individual bowl. Garnish with additional celery, cucumber, red bell peppers, jalapenos, and papaya. Swirl a spoonful of the orange papaya foam into each bowl of gazpacho.

Yields 4 to 5 servings

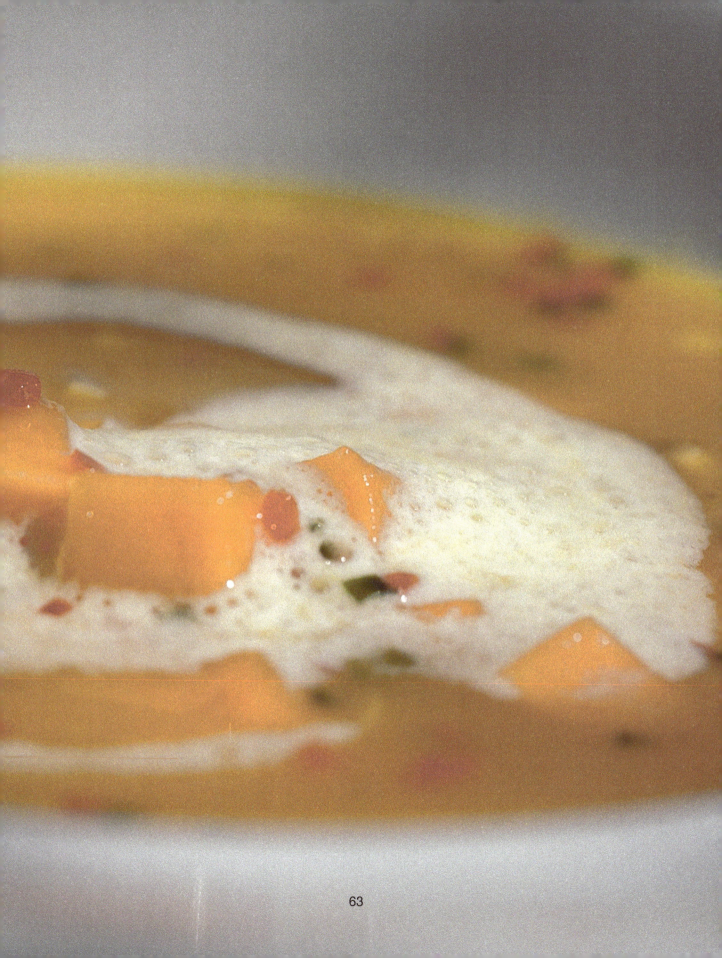

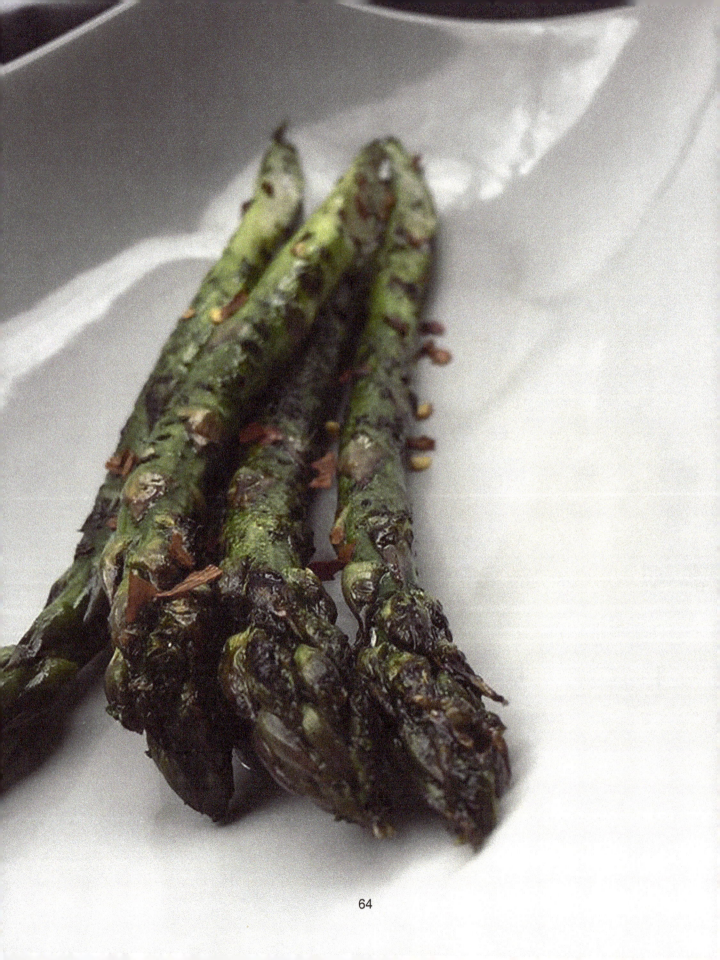

Grilled Asparagus with Herb Oil Marinade

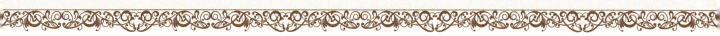

Ingredients:

1 ½ pounds of asparagus, trimmed
½ cup herb oil marinade (recipe on page 13)
salt and white pepper to taste

Instructions:

Preheat grill.

Trim stems (white parts) from the asparagus. Toss in herb oil marinade, salt, and pepper.

Spray grill with flavorless oil spray, and place marinated asparagus on grill. Turn after one minute, and cook for an additional 2 minutes until the asparagus are al dente (soft but firm).

Remove from the grill, and serve hot, at room temperature, or chilled for a topping on your favorite salad.

Yields 2 to 3 servings

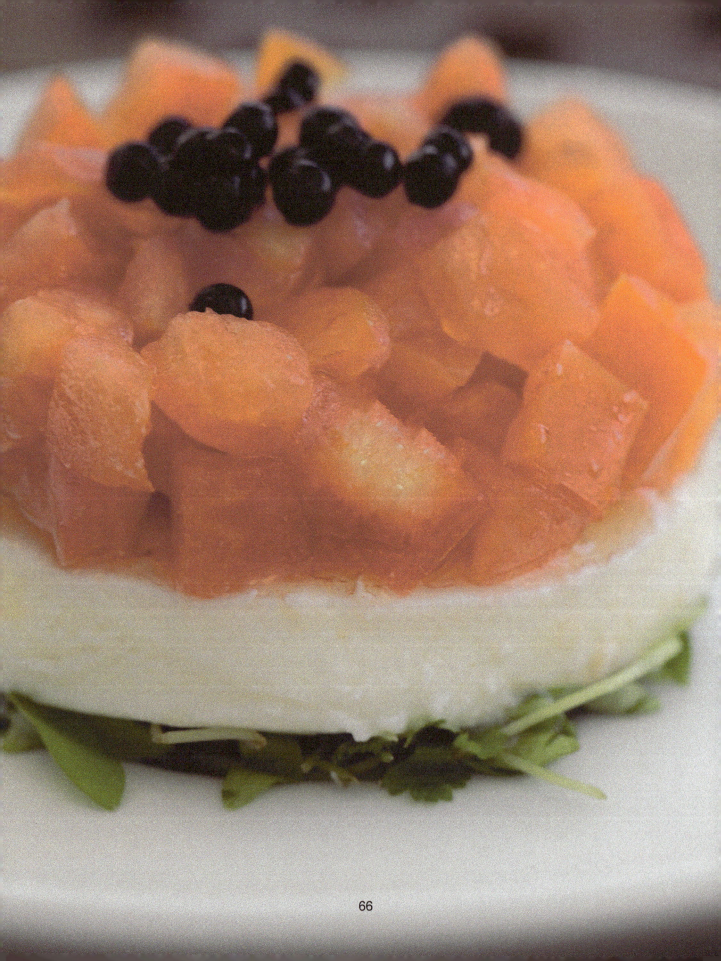

Tomato Concasse Caprese with Balsamic Pearls and Microgreens

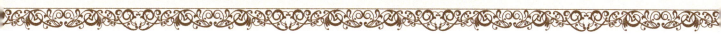

Ingredients:

8 ounces fresh mozzarella cheese

2 large tomatoes, concasse

1 cup micro greens of your choice (I used micro cilantro)

½ tablespoon freshly squeezed lemon juice

2 tablespoons of extra virgin olive oil

balsamic pearls (see recipe below) for garnish

balsamic glaze for garnish

Instructions:

Place a pot on the stove with 1 quart of salted water. Bring the water to a boil. Score tomatoes, and ladle the tomatoes gently into the water for approximately 1 to 2 minutes. Remove tomatoes from boiling water, and immediately immerse them into ice water.

After a couple of minutes, remove the tomatoes from the ice bath (the peel where the tomatoes have been scored should be peeling away from the flesh of the tomatoes).

Drain the tomatoes in a strainer. Cut the tomatoes in halves, and remove the seeds and veins. Next, dice the tomatoes into a small dice.

Place the tomatoes in a bowl, and toss with lemon juice, extra virgin olive oil, and salt and pepper to taste. Set aside to marinate.

Slice mozzarella cheese ball into half-inch rounds, and use a round ring mold to trim the edges so that you have a perfect round slice of mozzarella. Using a round mold, place the microgreens at the bottom of the mold. Next add the cheese and then the concasse of tomatoes. Gently slide the mold over the top of the salad, and garnish with balsamic pearls and balsamic glaze.

Yields 3 to 4 servings

*Balsamic Pearls

Ingredients:

⅔ cups balsamic vinegar
1 (1 ½–2 g) packages agar-agar, 10-sachet box
olive oil

Instructions:

Before starting, fill a tall glass with olive oil, and place it into the freezer for at least 30 minutes. The oil needs to be very cold so the balsamic vinegar pearls will cool before they reach the bottom. Once the oil is cold, you may continue making the balsamic vinegar pearls.

Add the balsamic vinegar to a pot along with the agar-agar, and bring to a boil while stirring. Once it begins to boil, remove it from the heat and let it cool slightly.

Drip the hot liquid using a dropper or syringe into the cold olive oil. It's best to try to leave drops of equal size, but you can always sort them into different sizes of balsamic vinegar pearls once they are done. Once all the pearls are made, you can remove them from the olive oil and rinse them in water.

*Recipe is from *Modernist Cooking*

Yields approximately 24 to 36 pearls

Jicama and Pomelo Salad

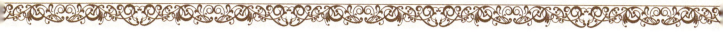

Ingredients:

- 2 tablespoons juice from about 2 limes, plus more to taste
- 2 tablespoons palm or brown sugar, plus more to taste
- 1 medium clove garlic, minced
- 2 teaspoons soy sauce
- 1 small red thai bird chili, finely sliced (optional)
- red pepper flakes, to taste, plus 3 to 4 whole dried red chilies, if desired
- 1 pomelo, segments removed and cut into 1-inch pieces
- 1 jicama bulb, peeled and cut into ½ by ½ by 2-inch batons
- 2 cups shredded napa cabbage
- 1 cup picked mung bean sprouts
- ¼ cups crushed roasted peanuts
- ½ cups rough chopped fresh cilantro leaves and tender stems
- 2 tablespoons store-bought or homemade Thai-style fried shallots

Instructions:

Combine lime juice, sugar, garlic, soy sauce, pepper flakes, 1 teaspoon dried chili, and whole dried chilies (if using) in a large bowl, and whisk until sugar is completely dissolved. Add pomelo, jicama, cabbage, sprouts, peanuts, and cilantro. Toss to combine, then season with more chili, lime juice, and sugar if desired.

Transfer to a serving platter, sprinkle with shallots, and serve.

Yields 3 to 4 servings

Thai Kale Salad

Ingredients:

- 4–5 cups packed curly kale
- 8 ounces firm tofu cut into 1 inch cubes
- ½ cups thinly sliced carrots
- 3 small radishes, thinly sliced (or substitute ¼ cups sliced red onion)
- ½ tablespoon sesame oil
- ½ tablespoon agave syrup
- 1 tablespoon sesame seeds
- 1 teaspoon lime juice
- 3–4 tablespoons peanut sauce for topping

Peanut Sauce:

- ¼ cups organic natural peanut butter
- 1 tablespoon soy sauce
- 2–3 tablespoons agave syrup
- juice of half a lime (1 ½ tablespoons)
- ½ teaspoons chili garlic sauce
- hot water
- optional: sriracha for a little heat

Instructions:

Drain tofu by wrapping in a towel and pressing gently. Let rest for 5 minutes. Then unwrap, cube, and toss in 1 tablespoon sesame seeds, and sear in hot pan over medium heat.

Prepare peanut sauce by whisking all ingredients together from peanut sauce ingredient list, except the water. Then add in 1 tablespoon very hot water a little at a time until pourable. Taste and adjust seasonings as needed.

Add kale to a large mixing bowl, and drizzle over 1 teaspoon lime juice and ½ tablespoons each toasted sesame oil and agave. Massage with hands for 1 minute to incorporate ingredients and soften the leaves.

Add kale to serving plate or bowl, and top with sliced radishes, carrot and sesame tofu. Drizzle with peanut sauce and serve immediately. Leftovers store well, even lightly dressed. Will keep refrigerated for up to a couple days, though best when fresh.

Watermelon, Feta, and Mint Caprese

Ingredients:

1 medium-sized seedless watermelon (rind removed and sliced in squares)

balsamic glaze

8 ounces of feta cheese, drained and sliced

fresh mint leaves

2 tablespoons of extra virgin olive oil

kosher sea salt

Instructions:

Cut watermelon in half, and cut the melon in 2inch slices. Place watermelon slices on cutting board, and using a chef's knife, slice the top and bottoms rinds off first and then both sides forming a square. Cut the squared slice into four even squares.

In a large mixing bowl, drizzle olive oil over the melon slices and sprinkle with sea salt. Remove melon slices from bowl, and place an individual slice on a plate. Top with feta, and then top with another melon slice. Complete the process again to have 3 slices of melon and 2 slices of feta.

Drizzle with the balsamic glaze, and garnish with mint leaves.

Yields 3 to 4 servings

Coconut Cauliflower Rice

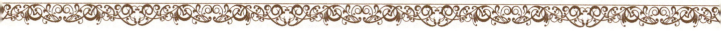

Ingredients:

- 1 tablespoon coconut oil
- 1 ¼ pound cauliflower florets
- 1 can full fat coconut milk
- 1 cup shredded coconut
- ¼ cups lime juice
- 4 teaspoons lime zest
- ½ cups fresh cilantro, minced

Instructions:

Add the coconut oil to a large pan over low-medium heat. While it is warming up, pulse the cauliflower florets in a food processor into rice-sized pieces.

Add the rice cauliflower to a sauté pan, and stir through to coat with the coconut oil. Cook for about 5 minutes to get rid of some the of the excess moisture in the cauliflower.

Stir in the coconut milk and shredded coconut. Add about three quarters of the lime juice. Bring to a simmer, and turn the heat down slightly so that the pan doesn't come to a boil. Simmer until tender and the liquid has been absorbed, about 10 minutes.

Pour in the last of the lime juice, along with the lime zest and fresh cilantro. Season to taste with salt. Stir through and cook until the lime juice has evaporated.

Yields 3 to 4 servings

Cauliflower Veloute with Wild Mushrooms and Balsamic Pearls

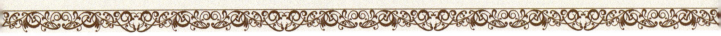

Ingredients:

1 tablespoon unsalted butter
1 tablespoon white truffle oil
1 medium shallot, chopped
1 large head cauliflower rough chopped
2 large russet potatoes medium dice
1 cup heavy cream
2 ¼ cups clear vegetable broth
2 tablespoons olive oil
sea salt and freshly ground black pepper to taste
8 ounces of fresh assortment of wild mushrooms
1 ounce balsamic pearls (see recipe on page 68)
fresh tarragon

Instructions:

Melt butter and truffle oil in a large pan over medium heat. Add shallot and sweat for about 6 minutes. Add the chopped cauliflower, diced potatoes, heavy cream, and vegetable broth to the cooked shallots. Reduce the heat to medium low, cover, and simmer for approximately 20 to 25 minutes.

In a separate pan, sauté mushrooms in 2 tablespoons of extra virgin olive oil over medium heat. Sauté until slightly caramelized.

After the cauliflower has cooked for allotted time and tenderness, blend on medium with a robot coup or blender. Blend the cauliflower mixture until it is smooth. Return mixture back to pan, and simmer for an additional 5 to 7 minutes. Place soup in bowl and garnish with morels, tarragon, and balsamic pearls.

Yields 3 to 4 servings

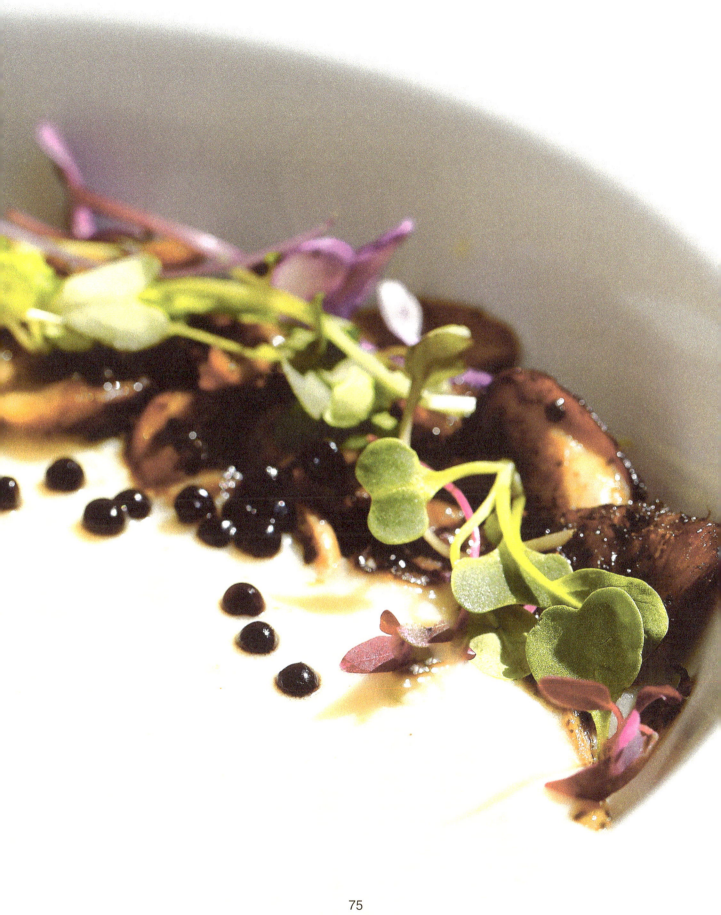

Ful Mudammas

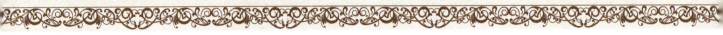

Ingredients:

- 1 pound dry fava beans
- 6 cups water (for soaking the beans) plus an additional 6 cups for cooking
- 2 beefsteak tomatoes, diced
- 1 red onion, chopped
- ½ cup cilantro, chopped
- 2 tablespoons of garlic paste
- 2 tablespoons of tahini
- 2 teaspoons kosher sea salt
- ¼ teaspoon white pepper
- juice of one medium freshly squeezed lemon
- 1 teaspoon plus ½ cup of extra virgin olive oil
- 2 jalapeno peppers chopped

Instructions:

Wash the beans, and boil for 10 minutes in salted water. Remove from heat, cover, and let the beans soak for one hour.

After the beans have soaked for an hour, drain the water and wash the beans. Place the beans in a 3-quart Dutch oven, and add all other ingredients.

Cook the beans over medium heat covered for one hour, stirring frequently so they don't scorch or stick to the bottom of the pot.

Approximately every 15 to 20 minutes. When the beans have cooked for about 45 minutes, take a wooden spoon and mash some of the beans to create a gravy or paste. Continue to cook the beans for an additional 15 minutes or until the beans are soft.

Yields 3 to 4 servings

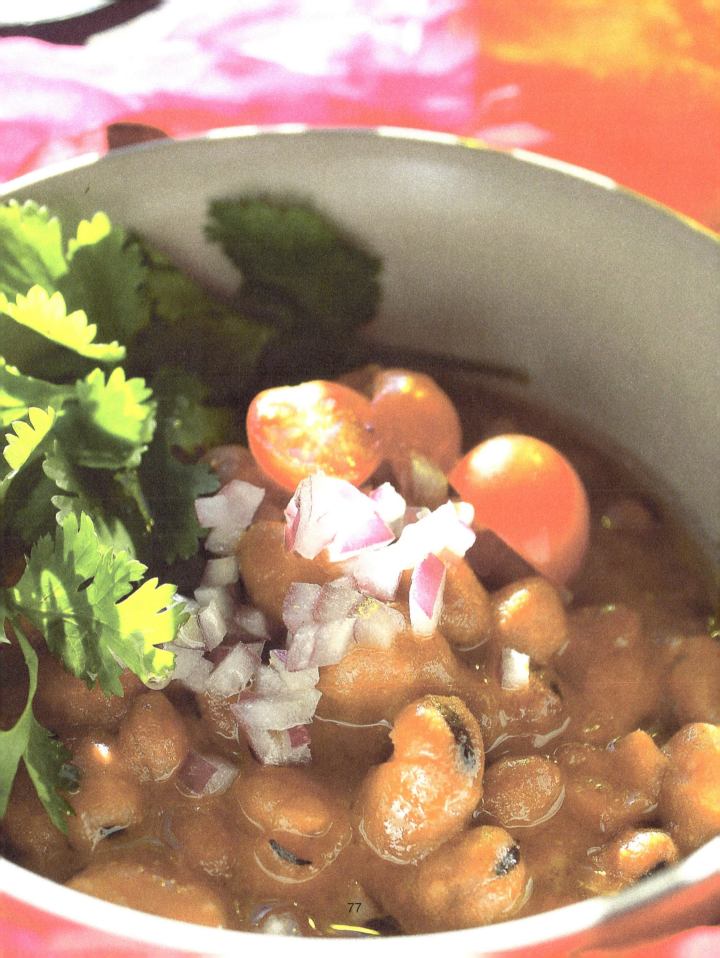

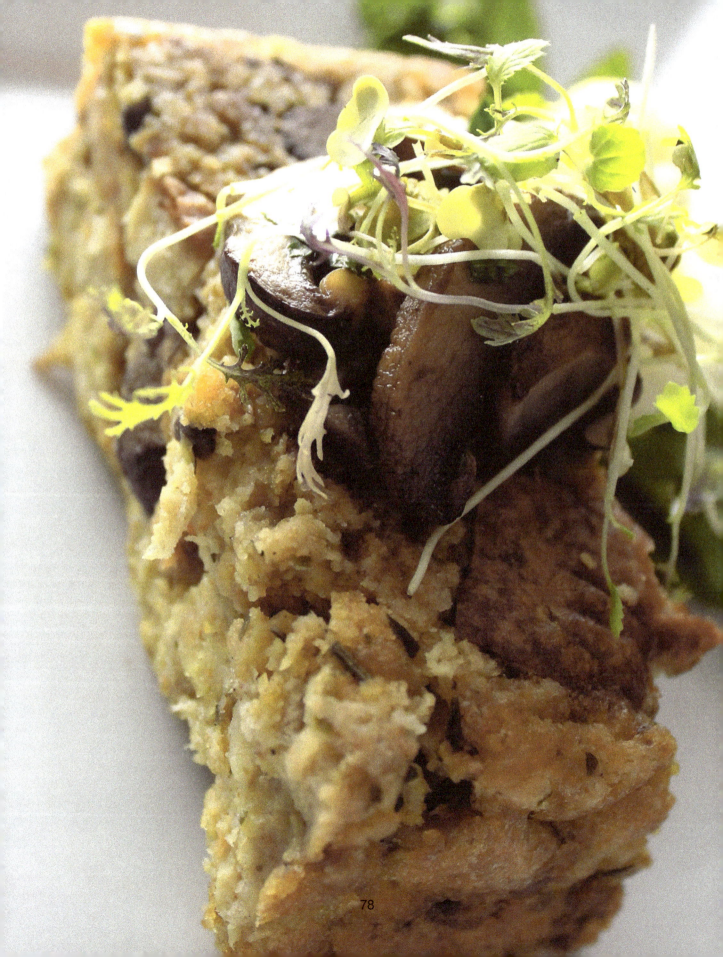

Savory Bread Pudding with Mushrooms

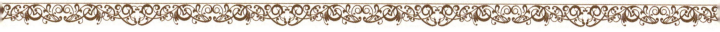

Ingredients:

- 2 day-old baguettes
- ¼ cups olive oil
- 4 teaspoons chopped fresh thyme
- 1 large garlic clove, minced
- 6 tablespoons (¾ stick) butter
- 1 pound assorted fresh mushrooms
- 1 ½ cups finely chopped onion
- 1 ½ cups thinly sliced celery
- 1 cup finely chopped green bell pepper
- ¼ cups chopped fresh parsley
- 3 ½ cups heavy whipping cream
- 2 teaspoons salt
- 1 teaspoon freshly ground black pepper
- ¼ cups finely grated parmesan cheese

Instructions:

Preheat oven to 375°F. Butter 13×9×2–inch glass baking dish.

Cut baguettes into 1-inch cubes. Place cubes in very large bowl. Add oil, thyme, and garlic; toss to coat.

Spread cubes out on large rimmed baking sheet. Sprinkle with salt and pepper. Bake until golden and slightly crunchy, stirring occasionally, about 20 minutes.

Return toasted bread cubes to same very large bowl.

Melt butter in large skillet over medium-high heat. Add mushrooms, onion, celery, and bell pepper. Sauté until soft and juices have evaporated, about 15 minutes. Add sautéed vegetables and parsley to bread cubes.

Whisk heavy cream, salt and ground pepper in large bowl. Mix custard into bread and vegetables. Transfer stuffing to prepared dish. Sprinkle cheese over.

Preheat oven to 350°F.

Bake stuffing uncovered until set and top is golden, about 1 hour. Let stand 15 minutes.

Yields 3 to 4 servings

Quinoa Salad with Cranberries and Spinach

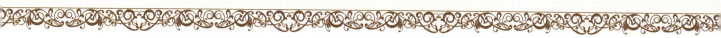

Ingredients:

½ cups uncooked quinoa

3 cups water

zest of 1 lemon *(grated)* juice of 2 lemons

1 tablespoon extra-virgin olive oil

salt and pepper to taste

2–3 large handfuls shredded spinach

½ cups of dried cranberries

Instructions:

Rinse your quinoa well. Add to a saucepan, and cover with the water.

Bring to the boil then cover with a lid and turn to the lowest possible setting.

Leave to cook for about 10 minutes or until all the water is absorbed.

Remove from heat.

Add the lemon zest to the hot quinoa. Stir and leave to cool.

Once quinoa is completely cool, add the lemon juice, olive oil, salt, and pepper to taste, and stir well.

Add the spinach and cranberries to the quinoa, and stir until well incorporated.

Yields 3 to 4 servings

Papa al Pomodoro (Tuscan Bread Soup)

Ingredients:

3 tablespoons extra virgin olive oil
1 small onion, chopped
1 garlic clove, thinly sliced
2 pounds tomatoes, peeled, seeded and chopped
¾ pound day-old Italian bread, rough sliced
2 cups water
1 cup fresh torn basil leaves
freshly ground black pepper
crumbled gorgonzola

Instructions:

In a 12-inch sauté pan, heat the olive oil over a medium-high flame until hot but not smoking. Add the onion and garlic, and sauté for a few minutes, until onion is translucent. Add chopped tomatoes and their juices, and bring to a boil. Reduce to a simmer, and let cook until the tomatoes begin to soften and break down, about 5 minutes.

Using a wooden spoon, add the stale bread chunks and water. Continue simmering until all the bread has absorbed as much liquid as possible, yielding a baby food–like consistency. Add the basil. Season to taste with pepper.

Let the soup continue simmering for 10 more minutes, then serve immediately in warmed soup bowls. Garnish to taste with gorgonzola.

Yields 3 to 4 servings

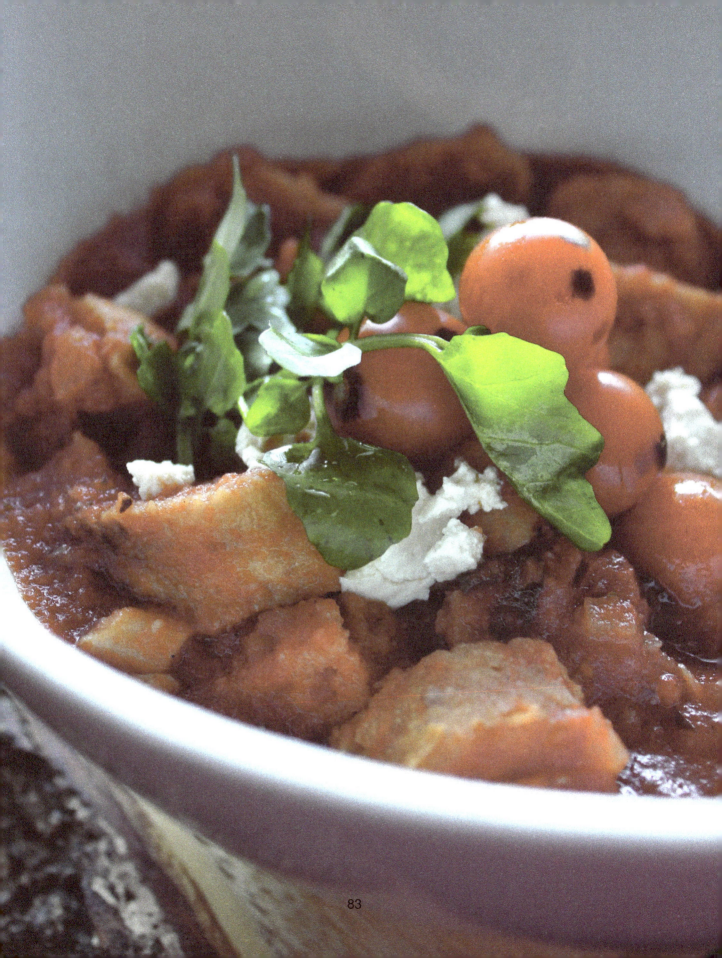

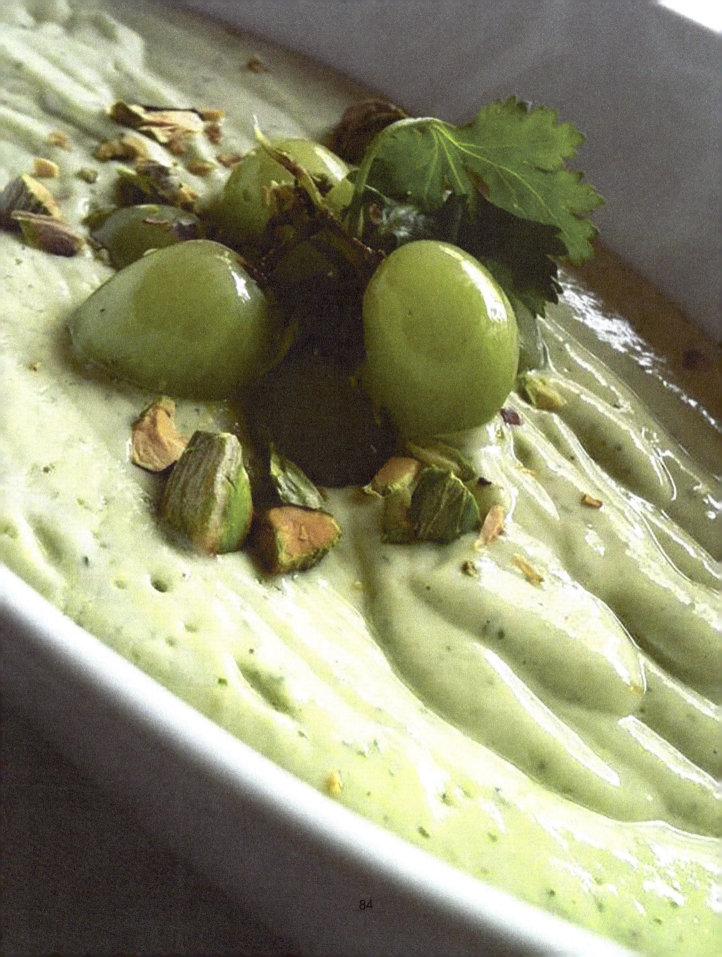

Chilled Avocado and Coconut Soup with Macerated Grapes

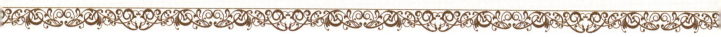

Ingredients:

1 medium avocado diced
1 tablespoon fresh lemon juice
¼ cup coarsely chopped fresh cilantro
1 teaspoon minced garlic
1 cup coconut milk
1 teaspoon kosher salt
¼ teaspoon freshly ground pepper
¼ teaspoon ground cumin
⅛ teaspoon cayenne pepper
¾ cup cold water
½ pound green grapes
½ cup limoncello

Instructions:

Place 1st 10 ingredients in food processor, starting with ½ cup water. Process until very smooth, about 1 minute, stopping once to scrape the sides of the owl with a spatula. Check consistency and, if desired, add up to ¼ cup more water and process to combine. Divide the avocado soup among 4 individual bowls. Refrigerate, covered, 30 minutes. Garnish with macerated grapes and cilantro, and serve.

Macerated Grapes

Prick grapes with a toothpick, and place them into a glass mixing bowl. Pour limoncello over grapes, cover, and refrigerate for at least 3 hours.

Yields 3 to 4 servings

Glazed Brussels Sprouts

Ingredients:

1 ½ pounds brussels sprouts, trimmed and cut in half through the core

¼ cups good olive oil

kosher salt and freshly ground black pepper

4 tablespoons balsamic glaze

Instructions:

Preheat oven to 400 degrees.

Place the brussels sprouts on a sheet pan, including some of the loose leaves, which get crispy when they're roasted. Add the olive oil, 1 ½ teaspoon salt, and ½ teaspoon pepper. Toss with your hands, and spread out in a single layer.

Roast the brussels sprouts for 20 to 30 minutes, until they're tender and nicely browned and the pancetta is cooked. Toss once during roasting.

Remove from the oven, drizzle immediately with the balsamic vinegar, and toss again. Taste for seasonings, and serve hot.

Yields 3 to 4 servings

Superfood Bowl with Fresh Kale, Brussels Sprouts, Quinoa, and Hempseeds with Green Goddess Dressing

Ingredients:

- 2 cups water
- 1 cup uncooked quinoa
- 1 cup brussels sprouts, cleaned and halved
- 1 packed cup kale, chopped
- extra virgin olive oil
- 2 tablespoons hempseeds

For the Green Goddess Dressing:

- 1 garlic clove
- 1 ½ small–medium avocados
- 5 tablespoons extra virgin olive oil
- 6 tablespoons water
- ¾ cups basil
- ¼ cups parsley
- ¼ cups chives
- ½ cups scallions (white parts removed)
- juice of 1 ½ small lemons
- 2 tablespoons apple cider vinegar
- ½ teaspoon salt

Instructions:

Bring water to a boil in a saucepan. Add quinoa, reduce heat to low, and cover. Simmer until all liquid has been absorbed, approximately 15–20 minutes, then fluff with a fork.

Toss brussels sprouts with olive oil and a pinch of sea salt. Roast in a 400-degree oven until slightly browned and crisp.

Add chopped kale to a small bowl, and drizzle with olive oil and a pinch of sea salt. Toss until kale is well coated with olive oil.

Green Goddess Dressing:

In a food processor, blend together the garlic, avocado, olive oil, and water. Add basil, parsley, chives, and scallions, and pulse to blend. Add lemon juice, apple cider vinegar, and salt, and blend to combine.

Arrange bowls with quinoa, brussels sprouts, kale, and hempseeds, and drizzle with desired amount of green goddess dressing.

Yields 3 to 4 servings

Vegan Causa (Peruvian Mashed Potato Salad)

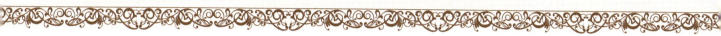

Ingredients:

6 pounds yellow flesh potatoes, peeled and quartered

1 ½ cups fresh lime juice

6 tablespoons extra virgin olive oil

4 tablespoons aji amarillo paste*

2 ½ tablespoons salt

12 ounces of seitan chickenless strips, chopped

4 ounces veganaise

3 cups yellow or red tomatoes, diced

½ cup black olives, pitted and chopped

24 each parsley sprigs

Instructions:

In saucepan, cook potatoes in 2 quarts of water for about 20 minutes. The potatoes should be soft but not mushy. Put the potatoes through a ricer, or mash with a potato masher.

Mix in lime juice, oil, aji amarillo paste, and salt.

Preheat another saucepan with 2 tablespoons of olive oil, and cook seitan chickenless strips over medium high heat. Sprinkle with salt and pepper, and cook for about 7 to 10 minutes. Remove from heat, and let cool.

In bowl, mix together seitan chickenless strips and veganaise.

Place 24 2-inch ring molds on plastic wrap–lined sheet pan. Spread ¼ cup potato mixture in bottom of 1 mold in even layer. Spread ¼ cup seitan mixture on top of potatoes in even layer; end with ¼ cup potato mixture.

Repeat with remaining ingredients to make 24 molds.

Refrigerate covered for at least 2 hours.

For each serving, to order: Invert 1 ring mold onto plate; carefully remove mold.

Garnish with 2 tablespoons tomatoes, 1 teaspoon olives and 1 parsley sprig.

Aji amarillo is a Peruvian hot yellow pepper that can be found puréed in jars or frozen whole. For whole aji amarillo, peel, seed and purée in a blender with a small amount of vegetable oil; use as directed.

Yields 24 servings

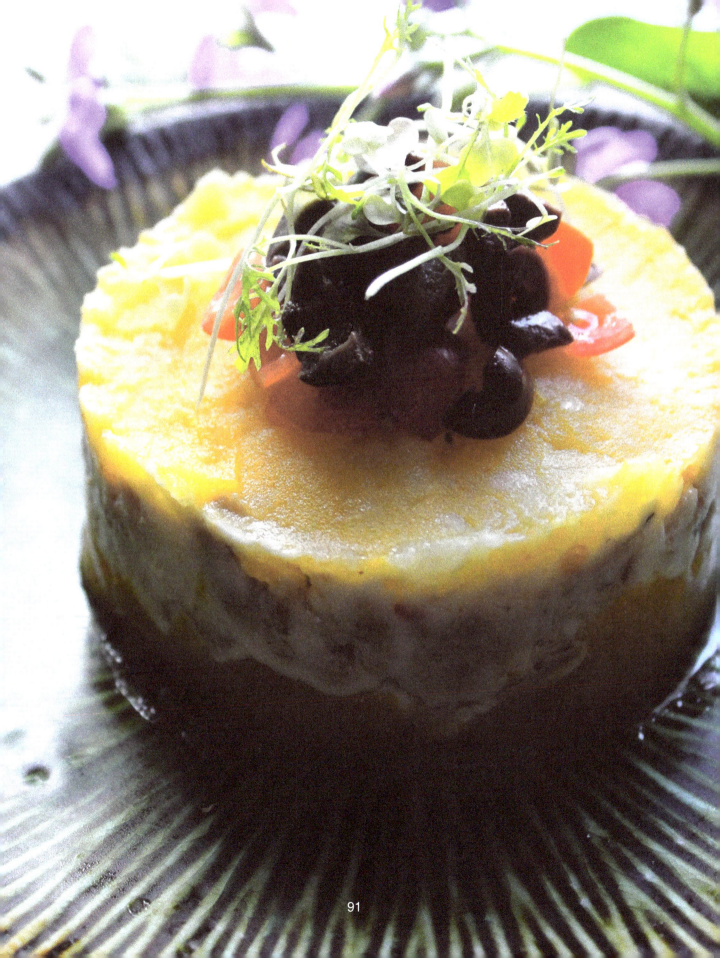

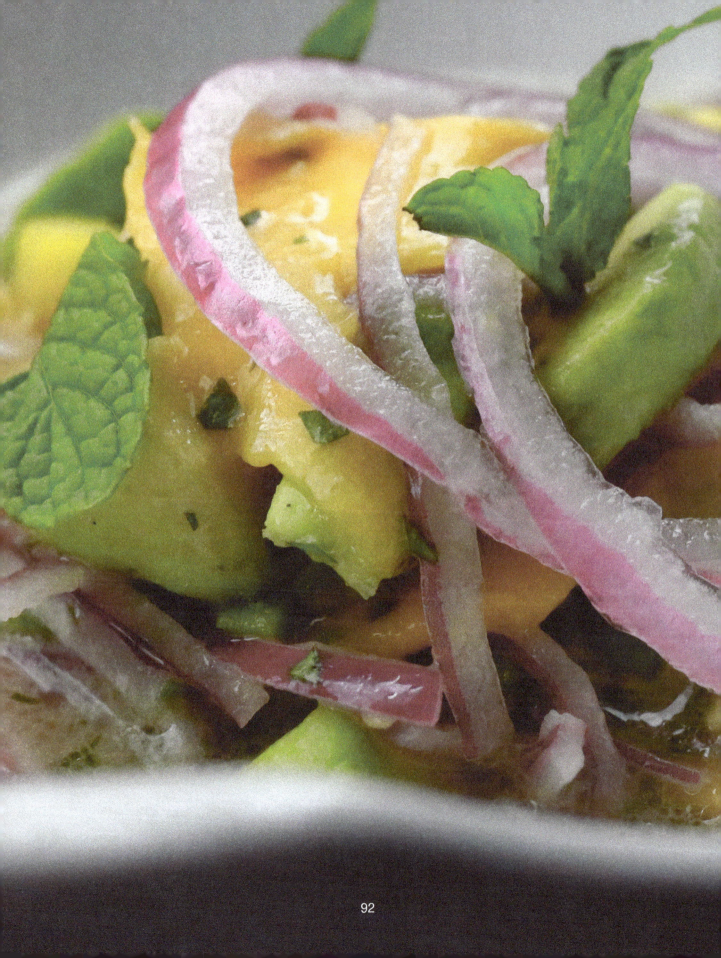

Mango and Avocado Ceviche

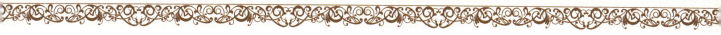

Ingredients:

1 large red onion, thinly sliced

2 mangoes, peeled and sliced1 large avocado, peeled and sliced

2 garlic cloves minced

juice of 4 limes

¼ teaspoons salt

1 Thai chili pepper, seeded and finely chopped

leaves from 2 cilantro sprigs, finely chopped

1 cup of coconut milk

Instructions:

Put the red onion in iced water for 10 minutes while you prepare the other ingredients.

Place the diced mangoes in a bowl, and add half the lime juice, coconut milk, and salt. Taste for balance, making sure it's not too sour.

Add the garlic and chili pepper, and then drain the onion and add it along with the cilantro leaves.

Stir everything gently to combine, and then leave in the fridge for 5 minutes to chill and marinate.

Serve in individual large glasses or bowls.

Yields 3 to 4 servings

Chapter 5

Main Dishes

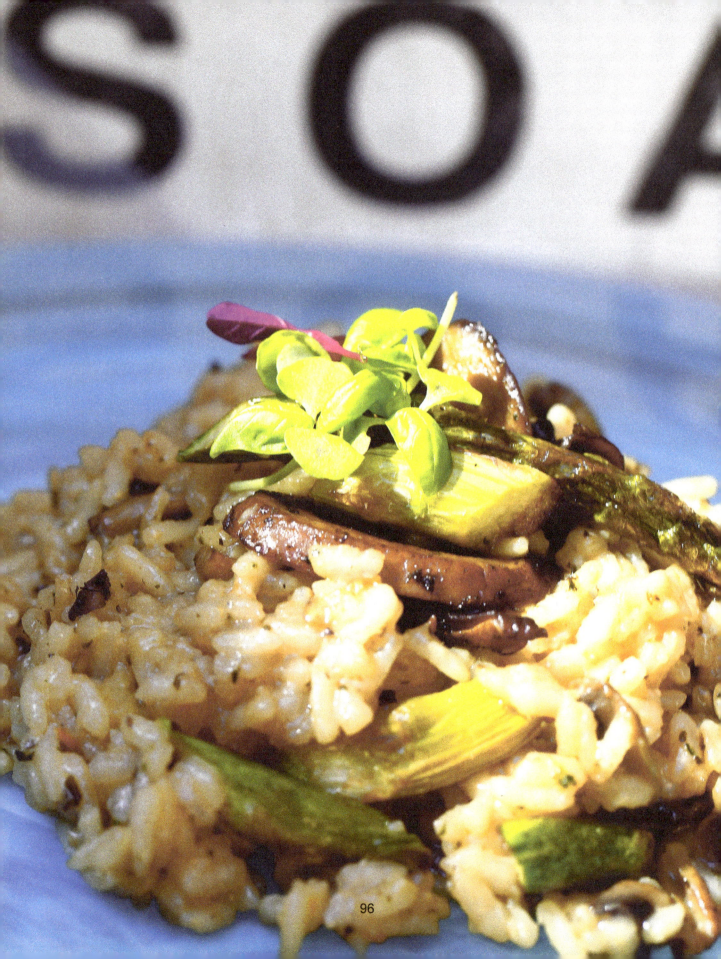

Risotto with Asparagus and Wild Mushrooms

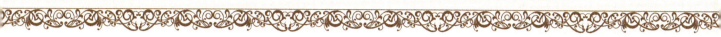

Ingredients:

- 1 pound green asparagus, trimmed and cut into 2-inch pieces
- ½ pound of assorted wild mushrooms
- 8 to 9 cups of blond vegetable stock
- ¼ cup extra-virgin olive oil
- ½ cup minced shallots
- 4 cloves of garlic, minced
- 3 cups carnaroli rice (arborio if you don't have carnaroli rice)
- 1 cup dry white wine
- 1 tablespoon vegan buttery spread
- salt and pepper to taste

Instructions:

Blanch asparagus in salted boiling water, until al dente (tender but firm). Remove from boiling water, and immerse in a bowl of ice-cold water.

Heat sauté pan over medium heat, and add the olive oil. Add the shallots, garlic, and cook until the onions are translucent, taking care not to burn the garlic. Add the wild fresh mushrooms and cook until softened, about 5 minutes.

Add the rice and stir until each grain is coated with oil and translucent. Continue to stir about 3 minutes. Add the wine, and stir until the wine is completely reduced.

Add the stock a ladle at a time, stirring frequently after each addition. Wait until the stock is completely reduced before adding the next ladle of stock. Make sure to reserve ¼ cup to add at the end.

When the rice is almost tender to the bit but slightly firm in the center and looks creamy (about 18 to 20 minutes), add the asparagus and a ladleful of stock. Continue to cook, stirring occasionally, until the asparagus is heated through and the rice is al dente.

Remove the risotto from the heat, and stir in the vegan buttery spread. Add reserved ¼ cup of stock. Season to taste with salt and pepper, and serve at once.

Yields 4 to 5 servings

Chickenless Mexican Stew

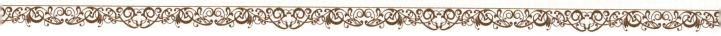

Ingredients:

1 tablespoon of blended oil
1 medium onion, small dice
1 ½ tablespoon of minced garlic
½ teaspoon dark brown sugar
1 teaspoon chipotle paste
1 8-ounce can chopped tomatoes
1 bag of Seitan chickenless strips
1 small red onion, sliced into rings
fresh coriander or cilantro leaves

Instructions:

Heat the oil in a medium saucepan. Add the onion, and cook for 5 minutes or until softened and starting to turn golden. Add the garlic after the onion has cooked. Stir in the sugar, chipotle paste, and tomatoes. Add the chickenless strips into the pan, spoon over the sauce, and simmer gently for 20 mins until the chicken has cooked.

Remove the chickenless strips from the pan and shred, then stir back into the sauce. Garnish with sliced red onion rings, the coriander, or cilantro, and serve with remaining red onion, tortillas, or rice.

Yields 4 to 5 servings

Curried Lentil Stew

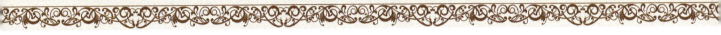

Ingredients:

4 tablespoons coconut oil
1 each onion, diced
1 each carrot, diced
2 celery ribs, diced
1 each fennel bulb, diced
1 each rutabaga, diced
2 each bell pepper, diced
3 each garlic clove, minced
4 tablespoons curry powder
2 tablespoons cayenne pepper (optional)
1 lime, zested (see note)
1 tablespoon kosher sea salt
1 pound dried red lentils
2 quarts blonde vegetable stock
1 cup coconut cream
1 bunch cilantro, chopped
1 lime, wedged
pomegranate molasses
steamed basmati rice (optional)

Instructions:

In a large heavy-bottomed pot, heat coconut oil. Add vegetables, and sauté for 10 minutes until lightly caramelized. Add curry powder and cayenne pepper. Stir until fragrant (approximately 30 seconds). Add lime zest, lentils, vegetable stock, and coconut cream.

Bring to a boil, and reduce to a simmer for approximately 20–30 minutes, until lentils and vegetables are tender.

Taste and adjust salt and cayenne pepper as desired.

Serve over steamed rice if desired with cilantro, lime, and pomegranate molasses.

Yields 4 to 5 servings

Creamy Saffron Risotto with Sautéed Brussels Sprouts and Chanterelles

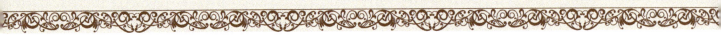

Ingredients:

2 ½ quarts light vegetable broth

2 tablespoons of extra virgin oil

4 tablespoons unsalted butter

1 medium onion, minced

1 large garlic clove minced

½ teaspoon saffron threads

3 ½ cups arborio rice

1 cup of shredded brussels sprouts

½ cup plus 2 tablespoons of coarsely chopped chanterelle mushrooms

1 ½ cups dry white wine

½ cup freshly grated parmigiano-reggiano cheese

salt and freshly ground pepper

¼ cup of heavy cream

Instructions:

In a large saucepan, bring the vegetable broth to a boil over high heat. Cover and keep hot over low heat.

Heat 2 tablespoons of extra virgin olive oil in a medium saucepan over medium-high heat. Add the onion and garlic, and cook, stirring occasionally, until softened, about 4 to 5 minutes. Add the rice, and stir to coat thoroughly and absorbed by the oil for approximately 2 minutes. Add the wine, and cook over moderately high heat, stirring until fully absorbed.

Add enough hot stock covering the rice one cup at a time, dissipating the liquid before adding additional liquid. Crumble in the saffron threads, and cook for 1 minute, constantly stirring.

Stir for about 2 minutes, and then add the butter, cheese, and heavy cream. Add the brussels sprouts and chanterelles, and cook the risotto for an additional 5 munutes

Season the risotto with salt and pepper and serve. Garnish with remaining brussels sprouts and chanterelles.

Yields 4 to 5 servings

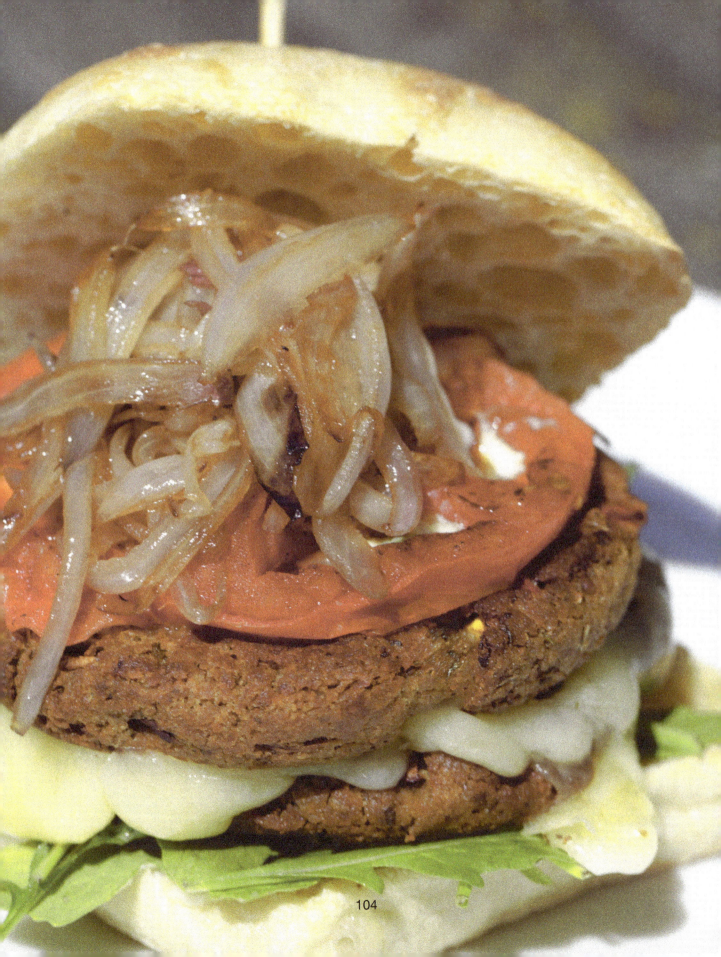

Chef Bev's Mushroom, Zucchini, and Yellow Squash Veggie Burgers

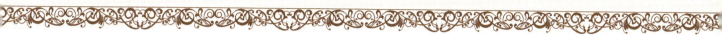

Ingredients:

1 cup of button mushroom, chopped

½ cup roasted zucchini, and yellow squash combined, chopped

1 medium roasted red, chopped

1 teaspoon onion powder

1 teaspoon garlic powder

2 slices of white bread, shredded and finely chopped

½ cup cento Italian bread crumbs

4 tablespoons Worcestershire sauce

1 dash of liquid smoke

2 tablespoons of canola oil for searing

Instructions:

Preheat oven to 350 degrees.

In a bowl, mix together chopped roasted zucchini, yellow squash, mushrooms, roasted red pepper, onion powder, and garlic powder. Add the chopped white bread, Italian bread crumbs, Worcestershire sauce, and liquid smoke. Mix well, making sure the mixture pulls away from the sides of the bowl and is not too sticky or too dry.

Form the mixture into 4 balls, and pat them to form patties. Set aside to rest for 5 to 7 minutes.

Next, heat oil in a sauté pan over medium-high heat.

Add the patties, and sear. Allow to sear for 2 minutes on each side. Turn off heat, and remove from pan.

Spray a sheet pan with cooking spray, and place veggie patties on the sheet pan, making sure they do not touch one another.

Place in a preheated oven and cook for 15 minutes, rotating the baking sheet halfway through the cooking process. Patties will be crisp on the inside and moist on the inside.

Serve on your favorite veggie burger bun, with your favorite toppings and condiments.

Yields 4 servings

Roasted Cauliflower Meuniere

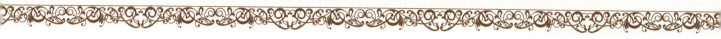

Ingredients:

1 large cauliflower, cut in thick slices
½ cups all-purpose flour
kosher salt and freshly ground black pepper
½ cup coconut milk
6 tablespoons unsalted butter
1 teaspoon grated lemon zest
6 tablespoons freshly squeezed lemon juice
1 tablespoon minced fresh parsley

Instructions:

Preheat the oven to 200 degrees. Have 2 heatproof dinner plates ready

Combine the flour, 2 teaspoons salt, and 1 teaspoon pepper in a large shallow plate. Soak the cauliflower slices in the coconut milk, and sprinkle with salt.

Heat 3 tablespoons of butter in a large (12-inch) sauté pan over medium heat until the butter begins to brown.

Dredge the cauliflower slices in the seasoned flour on both sides, and place them in the hot butter. Lower the heat to medium-low, and cook for 2 minutes.

Turn carefully with a metal spatula, and cook for 2 minutes on the other side. While the second side cooks, add ½ teaspoons of lemon zest and 3 tablespoons of lemon juice to the pan.

Carefully put the cauliflower slices on the ovenproof plates, and pour the sauce over them.

Place in a preheated oven and cook for 15 minutes, rotating the baking sheet halfway through the cooking process. Patties will be crisp on the outside and moist on the inside.

Yields 4 to 5 servings

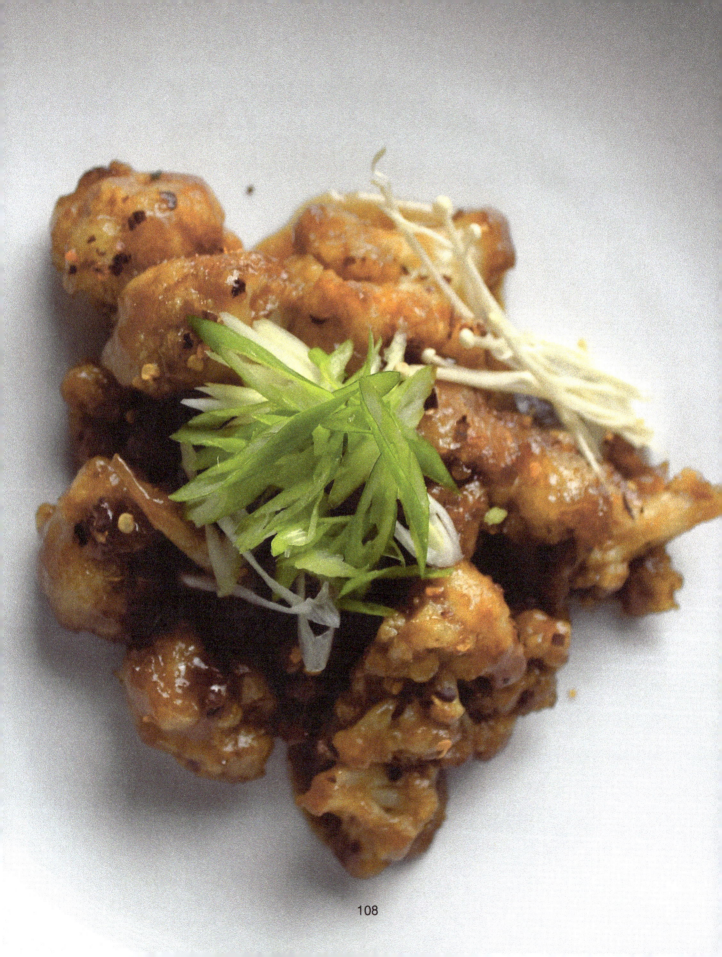

General Tzo's Cauliflower

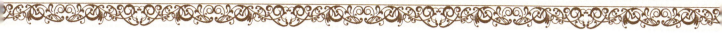

Ingredients:

1 cauliflower head, cut into florets

1 cup cornstarch

1 cup masa flour

grapeseed oil

Tzo's sauce (see below)

1 tablespoon coconut oil

1 tablespoon minced garlic

1 tablespoon minced ginger

1 chili pepper, sliced (optional)

½ cup tamari soy sauce

½ cup coconut sugar

¼ cup rice wine vinegar

½ cup coconut water

1 tablespoon cornstarch

3 tablespoons mirin

2 tablespoons Szechuan peppercorns, ground

4 each scallion, sharp bias cut

½ cup Chinese parsley, picked

Instructions:

To prepare sauce, heat coconut oil in a sauté pan over high heat. Add garlic and ginger (and optional chili pepper). Stir until fragrant, and immediately add soy sauce, sugar, vinegar, and coconut water to a boil. Reduce to a simmer.

Whisk together cornstarch and Mirin to create a slurry. Whisk into the sauce, and reduce sauce until of maple-syrup consistency.

Set aside Szechuan peppercorns, green onions, and Chinese parsley.

To prepare dish: steam cauliflower for 30 seconds to blanch the skin. Add to large mixing bowl, and toss to coat with cornstarch and masa flour.

Heat coconut oil in a wok to 325°F, and fry cauliflower until crispy and light golden brown (approximately 4 minutes).

Drain off excess oil, and toss to coat with sauce.

Plate over sticky rice, and top with peppercorns, scallions, and Chinese parsley.

Yields 4 to 5 servings

Chickenless Milano

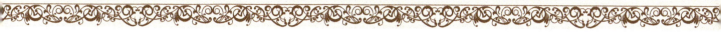

Ingredients:

- 2 tablespoons butter
- 2 cloves garlic minced
- ½ cup sun-dried tomatoes, chopped
- ½ cup chopped mushrooms
- 1 cup vegetable broth
- 1 cup heavy cream
- 2 cups Seitan chickenless strips
- salt and pepper to taste
- 2 tablespoons olive oil
- 2 tablespoons fresh basil
- 1 pound of linguini or penne pasta
- parmesan cheese

Instructions:

Heat a large skillet over medium heat; heat oil. Season chickenless strips with salt and pepper; cook until lightly golden about 3 to 5 minutes. Remove strips from heat, and set aside.

In the same skillet, melt butter over low heat with ¼ cup of the vegetable broth, scraping the pan to deglaze it. Add garlic, and cook briefly. Add the tomatoes and the remaining vegetable broth; increase heat to a boil. When you reach a boil, reduce to a simmer for about 10 minutes, leaving uncovered.

Serve with your favorite vegan or gluten-free pasta.

Yields 4 to 5 servings

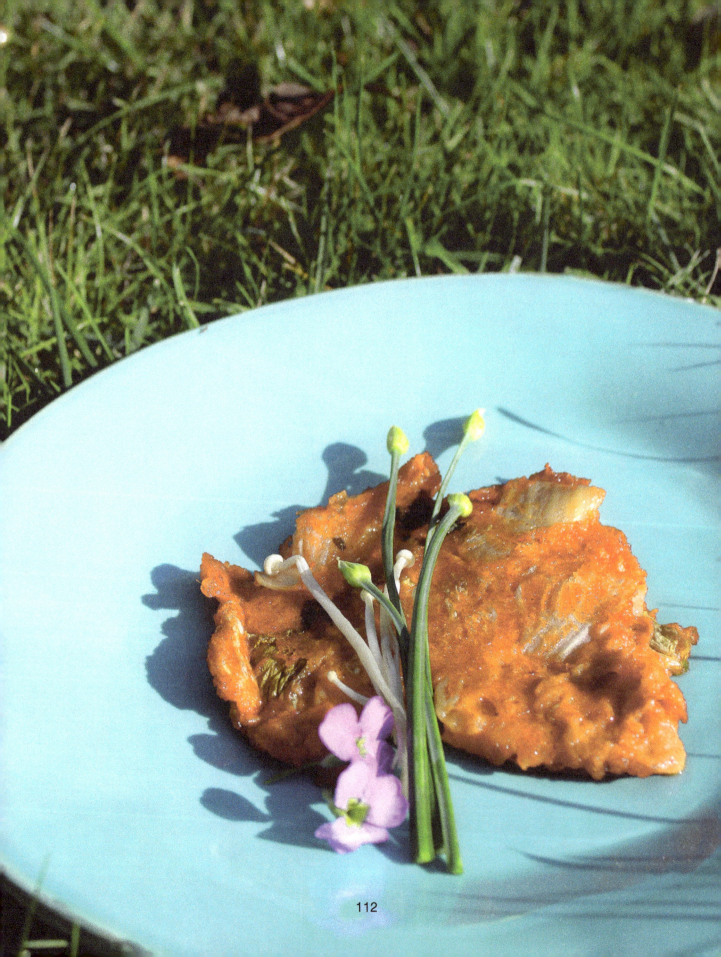

Kimchi Pancakes

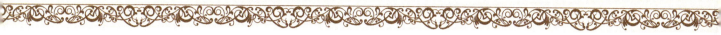

Ingredients:

- 1 cup chopped kimchi
- 3 tablespoons. kimchi juice
- 2 tablespoons. chopped scallions
- ½ teaspoon kosher sea salt
- ½ teaspoon pure cane sugar
- ¾ cup chickpea flour (garbanzo)
- ¼ cup water
- 2 tablespoons. sunflower oil

Instructions:

In a bowl, mix chopped kimchi, kimchi juice, chopped scallions, salt, sugar, chickpea flour, and water. Mix all ingredients well with a wooden spoon. Heat a 12-inch nonstick pan over medium-high heat, and drizzle about 2 tablespoons of sunflower oil.

Place the mixture of kimchi pancake batter on the pan, and spread it thinly and evenly with a spoon. Cook the pancake for 1–1 ½ minutes until the bottom becomes golden brown and crispy. After the bottom becomes brown, turn with a spatula and cook for an additional 1–1 ½ minutes.

Lower the heat to medium, and cook for another minute. Turn pancake once more, and cook for an additional 30 seconds before transferring to a serving plate.

Yields 4 to 5 servings

Braised Eggplant with Tofu in Garlic Sauce

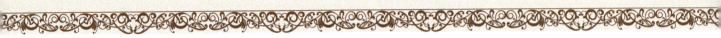

Ingredients:

- 2 pounds Chinese eggplant, cut 2-inch large dice
- 2 teaspoons mirin
- ¾ cups dry sherry
- 1 tablespoon corn starch
- 3 tablespoons soy sauce
- 2 tablespoons brown sugar
- 1 tablespoon Korean chili paste
- 1 tablespoon sesame oil
- 2 tablespoons vegetable oil
- 2 whole cloves garlic, plus 4 whole cloves garlic, thinly sliced
- 2 scallions, whites and greens thinly sliced and separated
- 1 pound firm silken tofu, 1 inch dice
- 2 to 3 tablespoons rough chopped fresh cilantro leaves

Instructions:

Place eggplant in a large bamboo steamer, and set over a wok filled with 2 inches of water. Bring to a boil over high heat, reduce to a simmer, cover steamer, and cook until eggplant is completely tender, about 10 minutes. Set aside.

Whisk vinegar, wine, and cornstarch together to make a slurry until the cornstarch has dissolved. Add soy sauce, brown sugar, chili paste, and sesame oil. Set aside.

Heat a wok over medium heat, and add oil and garlic cloves, turning garlic cloves occasionally until light golden brown and fragrant, about 5 minutes. Discard whole cloves then increase heat to high and heat oil until smoking. Add sliced garlic, scallion whites. Cook, stirring and tossing constantly until fragrant and just beginning to brown, about 1 minute. Stir sauce to reincorporate cornstarch, then add to wok, stirring constantly. Add eggplant and tofu, and fold occasionally until thick and glossy, about 5 minutes longer. Stir in scallion greens and cilantro, and serve immediately with white rice.

Yields 4 to 5 servings

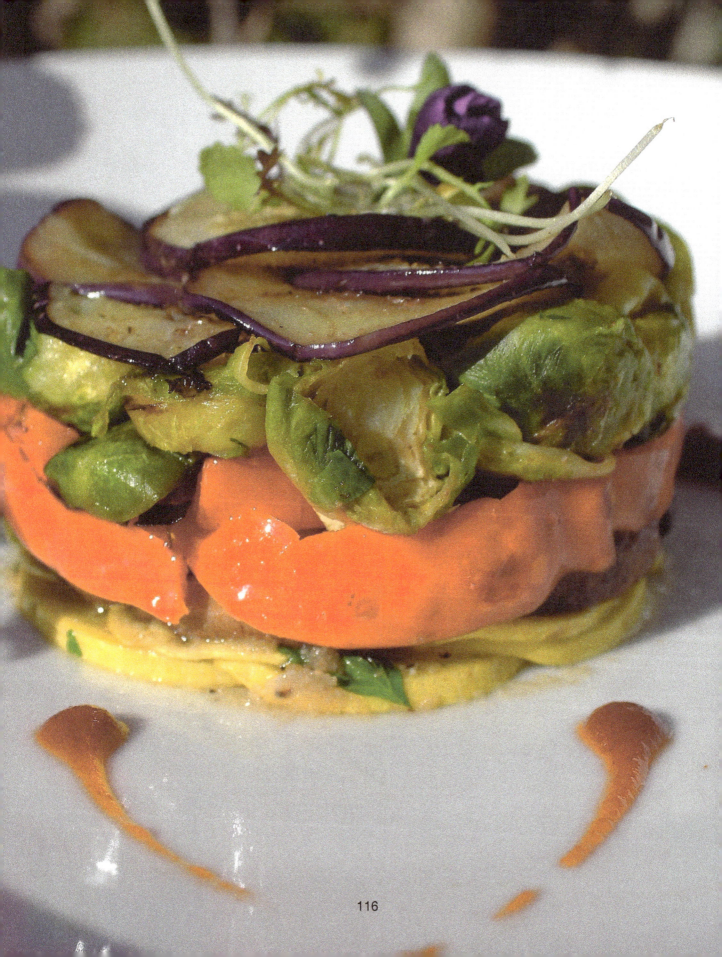

Ratatouille

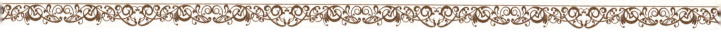

Ingredients:

1 ¼ ghee or olive oil
2 large yellow squash, sliced
1 Japanese eggplant, sliced
1 pound mushrooms, sliced thinly
1 large red pepper julienned
1 pound of brussel sprouts cut in half
9 garlic cloves
1 cup chopped parsley
½ pound chopped basil leaves
kosher sea salt

Instructions:

Sprinkle some sea salt on the eggplant slices, and put them in a colander in the kitchen sink. This step helps remove some of the moisture and bitterness in the eggplants.

Sauté mushrooms in 1 tablespoon of ghee or olive oil for about 10 munities with some seat until softened. Remove the mushrooms with slotted spoon, set aside, and cook the red peppers in the same manner with a little more oil or ghee.

Remove the red peppers with a slotted spoon, and repeat the process with the brussels sprouts, eggplant and squash, but for 6 minutes this time.

Remove red peppers, and set aside with the other vegetables. Remove the vegetables from the pan, and begin arranging them in individual 4 inch molds: squash first, then mushrooms, red peppers, brussels sprouts, and eggplant. Serve with your favorite red or white sauce.

Yields 4 to 5 servings

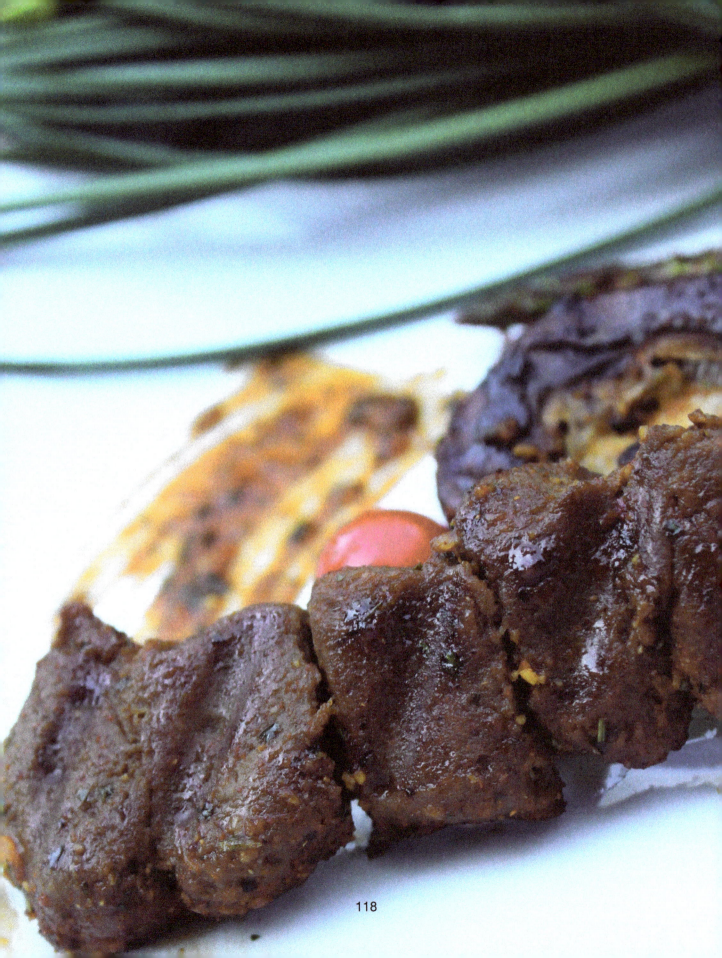

Moroccan Beefless Kebabs with Chermoula

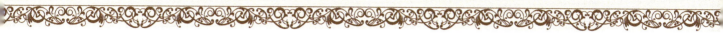

Ingredients:

1 cup of chermoula (recipe on page 17)
1 bag of Gardein beefless tips

Instructions:

Take the Gardein beefless tips and add the chermoula Sauce. Marinate for 20 to 30 minutes. Place the beefless tips on skewers. You can also add vegetables of your choice to the skewers. If using vegetables, alternate between the beefless tips and the vegetables on each skewer.

Heat a grill pan on medium, and coat it with olive oil. Grill the kebabs for 4 minutes on each side. Brush extra chermoula sauce over the kebabs, and cover to keep warm.

Serve with rice or your favorite grilled vegetables.

Yields 4 to 5 servings

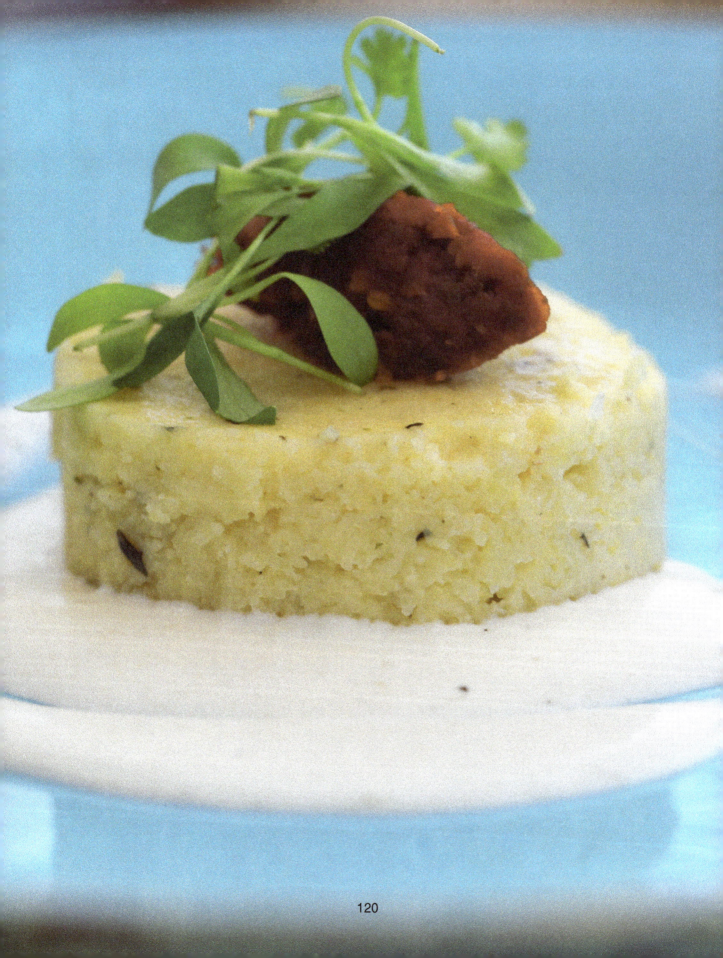

Gruyere Polenta Cakes with Sun-Dried Tomato Caper Quenelles and Alfredo Sauce

Ingredients:

- 2 cups polenta
- 3 cups boiling water
- 3 cups clear vegetable broth or water
- ½ cups coarsely chopped sun-dried tomatoes
- 1 tablespoon capers
- ¼ cup extra-virgin olive oil
- kosher sea salt
- 2 cups of grated gruyere
- 1½ ounces (3 tablespoons) unsalted butter, cut into 6 pieces
- 1 tablespoon. of dried Italian herbs
- freshly ground black pepper
- 1 quart heavy whipping cream
- 1 ½ cups alfredo sauce (recipe on page 30)
- microgreens to garnish

Instructions:

In a 4-quart saucepan, bring the water and broth to a boil. Whisk the broth and polenta together. Stir frequently to avoid lumps in the polenta. Bring to a boil over medium-high heat, whisking once or twice, about 5 minutes.

Turn the heat down to maintain a simmer, and continue cooking, whisking constantly, until the polenta thickens from soupy to porridgelike, about 2 minutes.

Turn the heat down to low. Cover and cook, stirring vigorously and scraping the bottom of the pan with a wooden spoon or spatula every couple of minutes. When you can see the bottom of the pan as you drag the spoon across it, 5 to 10 minutes later, begin tasting the polenta; it's done when it's thick, creamy, and tender. It should be granular but not gritty.

Remove from the heat, and stir in the cheese, butter, Italian herbs, heavy cream, and ½ teaspoon white pepper. Stir until the butter has melted. Place mixture into a deep baking dish, and set aside momentarily to set.

After the polenta has set for about 5 to 7 minutes, use a round ring mold to cut circles of polenta, which should be about 2 inches in thickness.

Sun-Dried Tomato Caper Quenelles

Using an immersion blender, blend together sundried tomatoes, capers, and olive oil. Blend ingredients until the mixture forms a tight paste. Using 2 small dinner teaspoons—not measuring teaspoons—measure about half of a teaspoon onto one of the spoons. Next, take the other teaspoon, and form a quenelle by scooping and molding the mixture through a pass of each spoon. Set the quenelles aside on a parchment-lined dish.

To assemble the polenta cakes, place a spoonful of alfredo on a plate, then the polenta cake. Next, place the tomato caper quenelle on top of the polenta cake, and garnish with microgreens.

Yields 4 to 5 servings

Dynamite Tofu

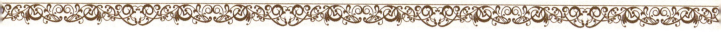

Ingredients:

1 pound extra-firm tofu, drained and cut into 1-inch cubes

¼ cups cornstarch

¼ cups sesame oil

¼ cups soy sauce or tamari

¼ cups hoisin sauce

1–2 tablespoons sriracha sauce, or to taste

1 tablespoon. agave nectar, or to taste

3 cloves garlic, minced

2 cups cooked rice

2 cups steamed or blanched broccoli

Instructions:

Preheat the oven to 400°F. Lightly coat the tofu cubes with the cornstarch. Place on a parchment-lined baking sheet, and bake for 20 minutes, or until golden.

Combine the sesame oil, soy sauce, hoisin sauce, Sriracha sauce, agave nectar, and garlic in a small bowl and mix. Add more Sriracha sauce or agave nectar if desired.

Place the baked tofu in a wok or pan on low heat. Add the sauce mixture, and stir until the tofu is coated and the sauce is heated through. Toss in the broccoli, and serve with cooked rice.

Yields 4 to 5 servings

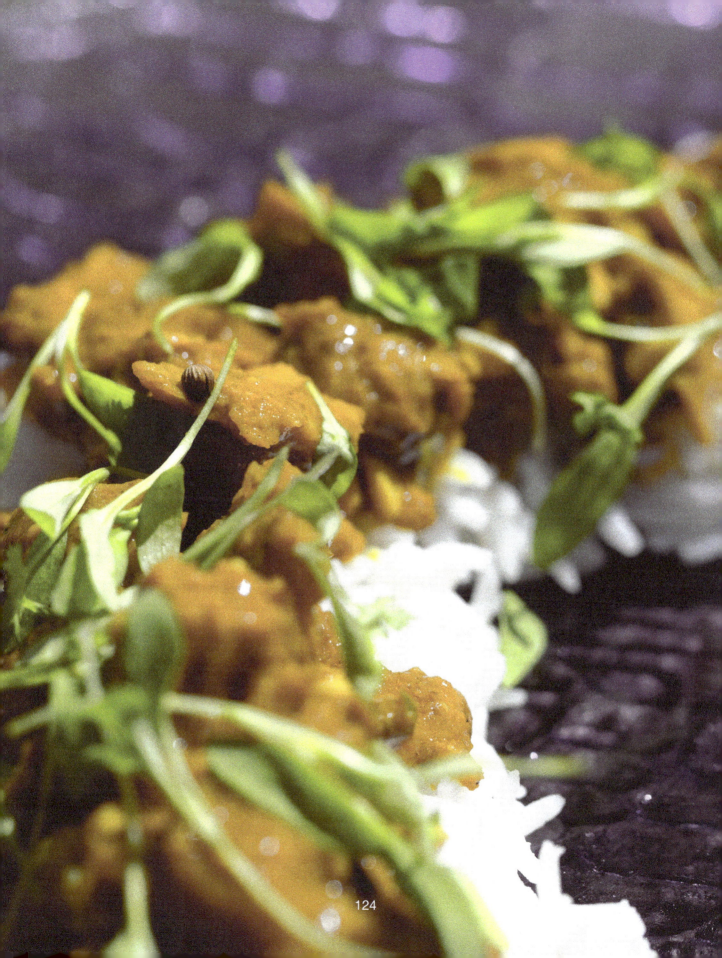

Butter Curry Seitan

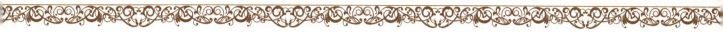

Ingredients:

- 1 pound seitan chickenless strips
- 1 red onion diced
- 3 tablespoons coconut oil
- 6 ounces can tomato paste
- ½ can coconut milk
- ½ tablespoon crushed garlic
- ½ teaspoon cardamom powder
- ½ teaspoon coriander powder
- 1 teaspoon fenugreek powder
- 1 teaspoon chili powder
- 1 teaspoon sea salt
- 4 tablespoons ghee (clarified butter)

Instructions:

In a large skillet or soup pot, heat the coconut oil over medium heat, and add the diced onion and sauté until translucent. Turn your heat down to low, and to the onion-and-oil mixture, add the crushed garlic, cardamom, coriander, fenugreek, and chili powder, and stir well to make a paste. Add the tomato paste to the onions and spices, and stir; this mixture will be very thick.

Turn your heat back up to medium, and add the coconut milk and salt. Use a whisk to blend the tomato paste spice mixture and coconut milk together into a thick sauce. Bring the sauce to a simmer, and add the seitan. Return the sauce and seitan to a simmer, turn down heat to medium low, cover, and cook for approximately 15 minutes or until the seitan is tender. Make sure you stir occasionally during the cooking process.

Yields 4 to 5 servings

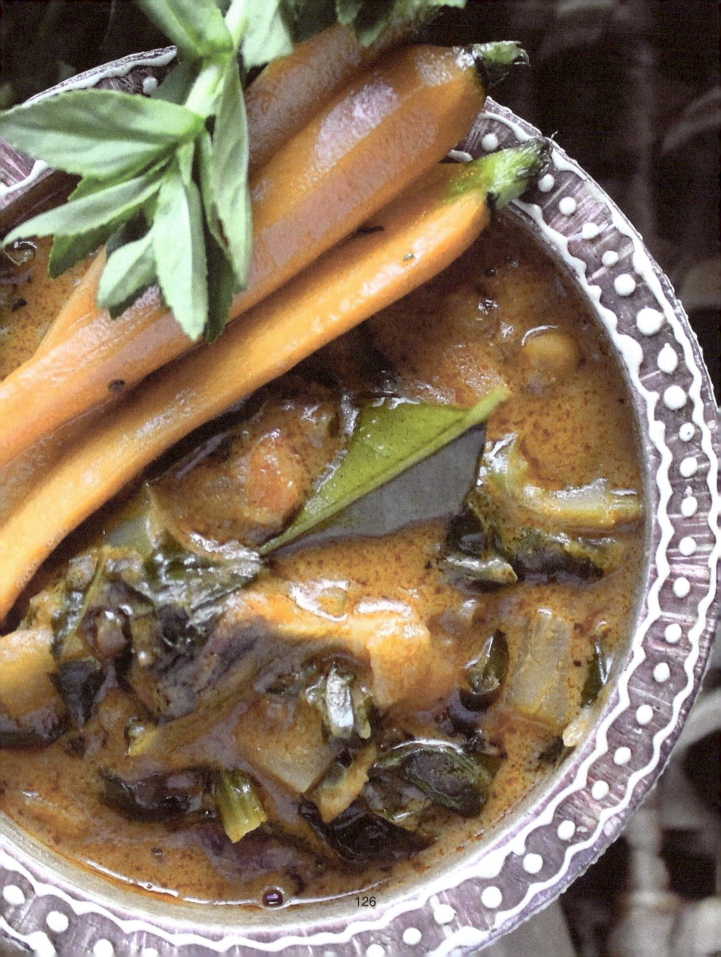

Ground Nut Stew

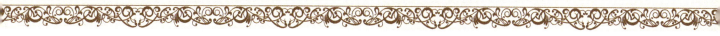

Ingredients:

1 tablespoon safflower oil
4 cloves garlic
1 inch fresh ginger
1 medium white yam, medium dice
1 medium onion, diced
½ cup chopped dates
1 teaspoon cumin
1 chipotle pepper in adobo sauce, finely chopped
1 6-ounce can tomato paste
½ cup natural style chunky peanut butter
6 cups vegetable broth
2 cups of collard greens
¼ bunch cilantro to garnish
chopped unsalted roasted peanuts to garnish
blanched heirloom carrots for garnish

Instructions:

Add safflower oil to a sauté pan over medium heat, and sauté garlic and ginger for about 2 minutes, making sure not to brown the garlic as it will become bitter. Add the diced onion, and sweat the onion until it becomes soft and translucent.

Next, add the diced yam, and continue cooking for 5 to 7 minutes more. Add the chipotle pepper, cumin, and tomato paste. Cook until the mixture is thoroughly combined. Add the peanut butter and vegetable broth, stirring frequently to allow the ingredients to become incorporated and are evenly combined. The sauce will appear thick.

Cover the pot, and increase the heat to medium high. Add the collard greens, and reduce the heat to medium low. Continue to cook the stew uncovered for approximately 15 minutes until the collards and yams have become soft.

Mash some of the yams against the pot with the back of a wooden spoon in order to thicken the stew. Add salt and pepper to taste, and garnish with cilantro leaves and chopped peanuts.

Yields 4 to 5 servings

Cauliflower Piccata

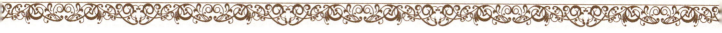

Ingredients:

- 1 head cauliflower
- 2 tablespoons vegetable oil, such as olive oil, grapeseed oil
- ¼ cup sliced leeks, white parts only
- ¼ cup shallots, minced
- 2 cloves garlic, minced
- ½ teaspoon salt
- ¼ teaspoon ground black pepper
- ¼ cup white wine
- ¼ cup capers
- ½ vegetable broth
- 2 teaspoons arrowroot
- ¼ cups lemon juice
- ¼ cups loosely packed parsley leaves, minced

Instructions:

Heat oven to 375ºF.

Remove outer green leaves and bottom portion of stem from cauliflower head. Slice the head vertically down through the center. Cut two 1-inch-thick slabs from each half.

On a sheet tray lined with parchment paper or aluminum foil, place cauliflower slabs. Drizzle with olive oil, and season with salt and pepper. Roast cauliflower for 15–20 minutes until edges begin to brown.

Meanwhile, as cauliflower roasts, sauté leeks, shallots, and garlic with salt and pepper in oil for 2–3 minutes. Deglaze the pan with white wine, and continue to cook until most of the wine has evaporated.

Stir arrowroot into vegetable broth to dissolve, and add to pan along with capers and lemon juice. Continue to cook for several minutes more until sauce thickens. Season with parsley.

To serve, place some sauce on the plate, and lay a roasted cauliflower slab over sauce. Spoon more sauce over the top of the cauliflower, and garnish with lemon slices and more minced parsley.

Yields 4 to 5 servings

Mushroom Pear Ragout

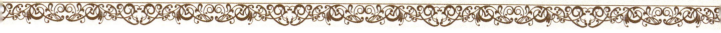

Ingredients:

½ cup of dry red wine

2.5 ounces of cremini mushrooms, diced

1 tablespoon of flour

½ cup unsalted butter

8 ounces white button mushrooms, diced

1 large pear (do not peel), diced

1 small sprig of thyme plus additional for garnish

1 pinch of dried sage

1 medium diced onions

2 level tablespoons of tomato paste

2 cloves peeled garlic

1 pint of vegetable stock

1 small bay leaf

Instructions:

Rinse off the mushrooms, and drain them on paper towels.

Heat the vegetable stock, add the tomato paste and red wine, and gently simmer. Add the thyme, peeled garlic, bay leaf, and sage to the stock.

In a separate thick-bottomes saucepan, melt the butter and add the onions and cook for about 3 to 4 minutes until they are soft, add the mushrooms and diced pears and cook for another 1 to 2 minutes. Gradually sprinkle in the flour and reduce heat to medium. Cook for the mixture until smooth, and there are no lumps from the flour.

Ladle the stock into the ragout and roux mixture, constantly whisking to avoid lumps.

Yields 3 to 4 servings

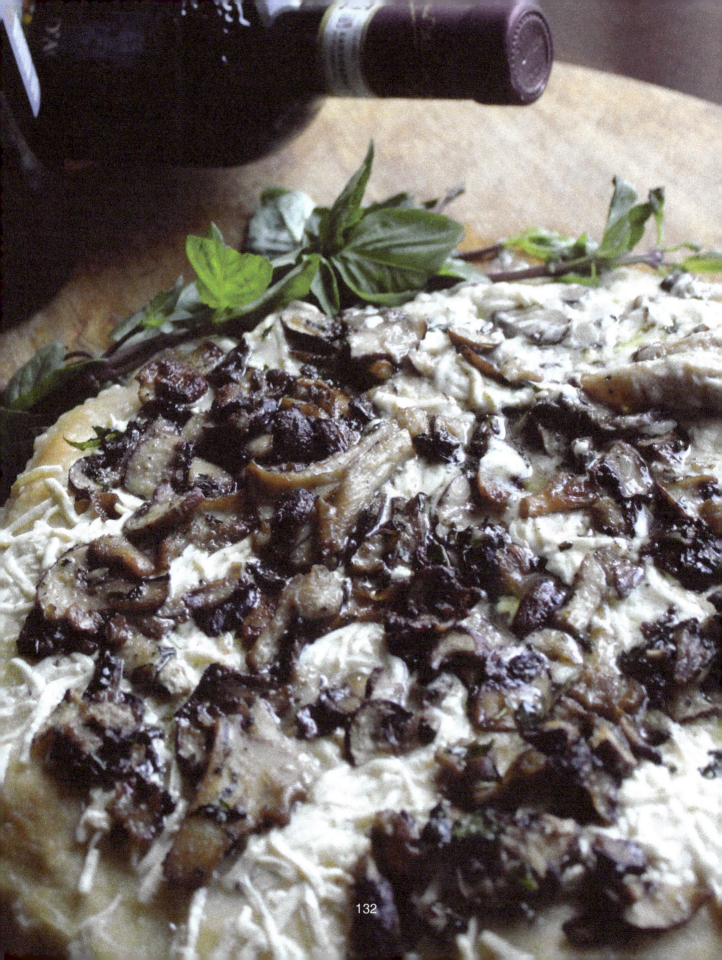

Wild Mushroom Pizza with Alfredo Sauce

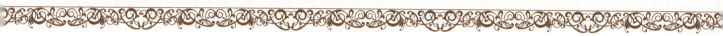

Ingredients:

    12-inch pizza crust
    1 ½ cup alfredo sauce (recipe on page 30)
    8 ounces of wild field mushrooms
    16 ounces of shredded mozzarella cheese (I used Daiya vegan mozzarella shreds)
    2 tablespoons of extra virgin olive oil
    1 tablespoon fresh oregano, chopped
    Pinch of white pepper

Pizza Crust

    2 ¼ teaspoons active dry yeast
    1 teaspoon honey (or agave)
    1 cup warm water
    2 ½ cups unbleached bread flour
    2 tablespoons olive oil
    1 teaspoon salt

Instructions:

Dissolve the yeast in the warm water in a medium bowl. Stir in the honey. Let it sit for about 10 minutes.

The yeast will be bubbly. Stir in the flour, olive oil, and salt. Beat until well combined. Let it rest for 5 minutes.

Put the dough on a lightly floured bowl. The dough will be quite sticky. Flour your hands, and knead the dough for just a few minutes. Put the dough on a piece of parchment, and put flour on your hands to press it out into a 12-inch round.

Assembling Pizza

Heat 2 tablespoons of extra virgin olive oil over medium heat, and add field mushrooms and fresh oregano. Add a pinch of white pepper, and continue cooking over medium heat for about 5 minutes.

Remove saucepan from heat, and remove mushrooms with a slotted spoon.

Preheat oven to 425 degrees. Place pizza dough on baking stone, and brush with extra virgin olive oil.

Ladle the white sauce onto the pizza dough, circling the ladle to take the sauce out to the edges. Add the mozzarella cheese, and top with the sautéed mushrooms and oregano.

Bake pizza pie for approximately 15 minutes until the cheese and the crust are golden brown.

Yields 8 slices

Roasted Eggplant Masala (Baingan Bharta)

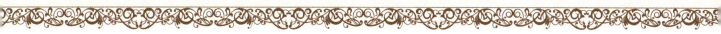

Ingredients:

1 large eggplant
1 red onion, small dice
1 teaspoon of garlic ginger paste
2 thai chili peppers, minced
2 medium tomatoes, small dice
¼ teaspoon turmeric powder
½ teaspoon red chili powder
¼ teaspoon garam masala
¼ teaspoon coriander
1 teaspoon lime juice
1 teaspoon turbinado sugar
2 tablespoons of cilantro chopped
2 tablespoons of mustard oil
salt and pepper to taste

Instructions:

Using a fork, prick the eggplant all over to allow the steam to escape while the eggplant is roasting. Coat the eggplant with a little oil, and salt and roast over an open flame or place in a 400-degree preheated oven and cook for about 30 minutes until the skin begins to separate from the flesh of the eggplant.

Allow the eggplant to cool for 5–10 minutes. Peel the charred skin from the eggplant, and mash the inside flesh using a potato masher or whisk. Place the mashed eggplant to the side.

Heat 2 tablespoons of mustard oil in a pan. Add chopped onion, and sauté until it turns translucent or soft and you can almost see through it. Add ginger-garlic paste, chopped red onion, and minced chili peppers. Sauté over medium heat for 2 minutes.

Add the chopped tomatoes to the onion mixture, and cook until soft. Add the turmeric powder, garam masala, coriander, and red chili powder to the mixture, and mix well. Mix in the mashed eggplant, sugar, lime juice, and salt, and cook over medium flame for 5 to 7 minutes.

Remove from heat, and garnish with chopped cilantro leaves or dried fenugreek.

Yields 4 to 5 servings

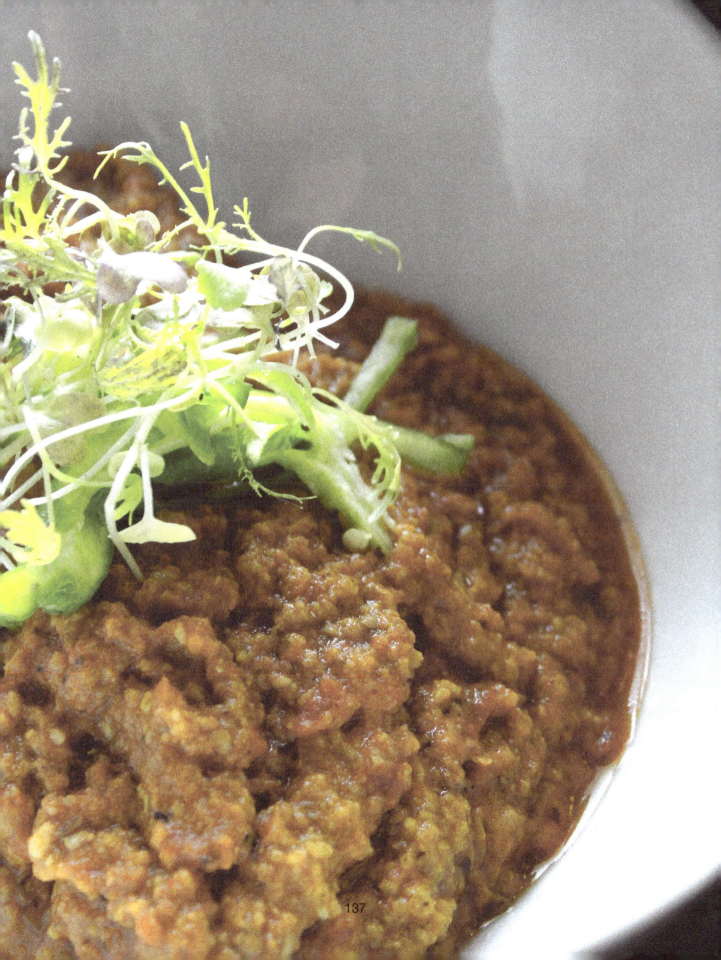

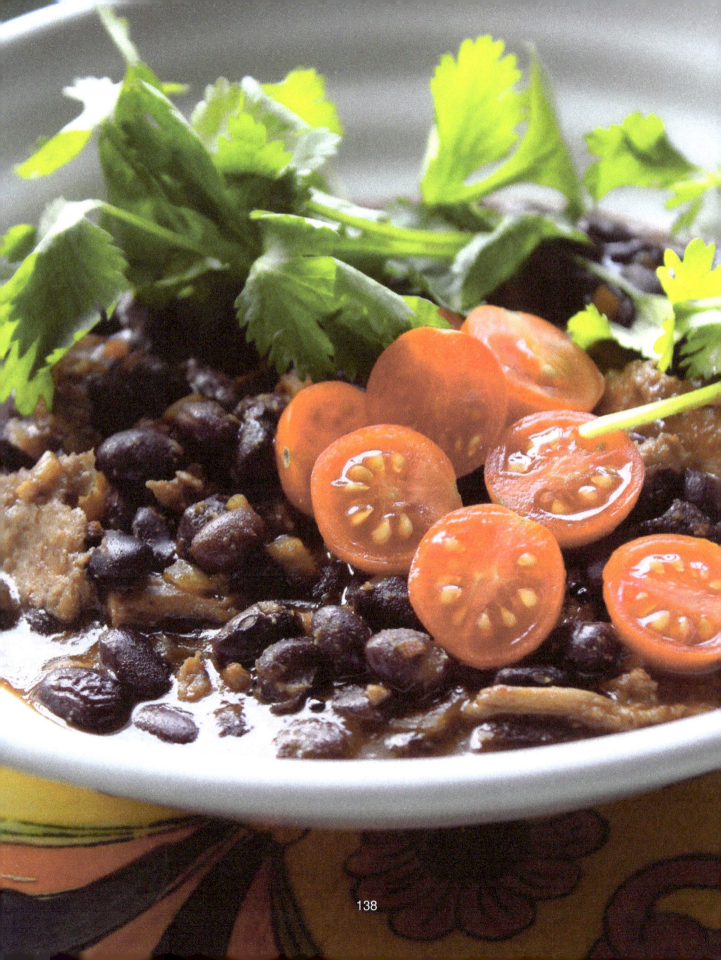

Easy Feijoada

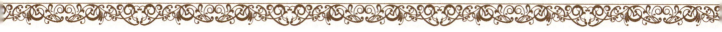

Ingredients:

½ tablespoon olive oil

1 package of smoked tempeh chopped

1 chopped smoked chipotle pepper in adobo

1 small onion, chopped finely

1 small carrot, peeled and chopped finely

1 green or red bell pepper, chopped finely

2 cloves garlic, minced

1 vegetable bouillon cube

2 teaspoons cumin powder

1 teaspoon paprika

1 teaspoon dried oregano or Italian seasoning

15 ounces can of black beans, drained and rinsed

3 cups water

½ cup of orange juice

salt and pepper to taste

Instructions:

In a medium saucepan, heat ½ tablespoon olive oil. Add onion, carrots, chipotle peppers, and bell pepper. Sauté on medium heat till the vegetables are soft, about 5 minutes.

Add minced garlic, and stir 30 seconds. Add the tempeh, cumin, paprika, vegetable bullion, orange juice and oregano. Stir for about 1 minute. Add the black beans, water and salt. Bring the stew to a boil. Then reduce heat to low, and simmer uncovered for about 30 minutes or until most of the liquid has evaporated. Mash some of the black beans using the back of a wooden spoon. Add the reserved tempeh, and cook another 5 minutes. Serve hot, and garnish with cilantro and heirloom grape tomatoes.

Yields 4 to 5 servings

Vegan Bolognese

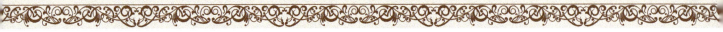

Ingredients:

- 2 tablespoons extra virgin olive oil
- 1 medium onion, diced
- 1 carrot, diced
- 1 tablespoon dried basil
- 1 tablespoon dried oregano
- 1 tablespoon dried thyme
- 1 teaspoon crushed red pepper flakes
- salt and pepper to taste
- 1 cup TVP (textured vegetable protein) (*Do not rehydrate.)
- ½ cup clear vegetable broth
- 16 ounces (2 cups) Chef Bev's sun-dried tomato and roasted garlic sauce (recipe on page 34)

Instructions:

In a large Dutch oven, heat the olive oil over medium heat. Add the chopped onions and carrots, and saute for about 7 minutes, until they begin to soften.

Add salt and pepper, basil, oregano, thyme, and crushed red pepper. Continue stirring the mixture over medium heat until fragrant. Next, add the TVP to the mixture and ½ cup vegetable broth, and then add the pasta sauce, stirring frequently to avoid scorching.

Reduce heat to medium low, and continue cooking the sauce mixture for about 15 minutes until TVP has rehydrated and the sauce has thickened.

Serve with your favorite vegan pasta.

Yields 4 to 5 servings

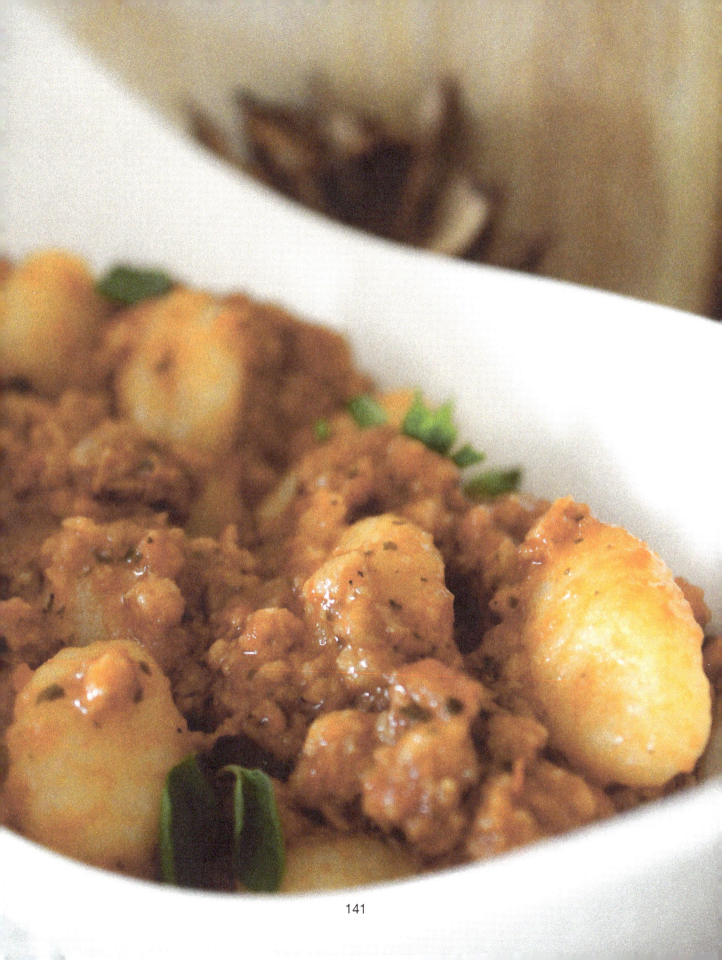

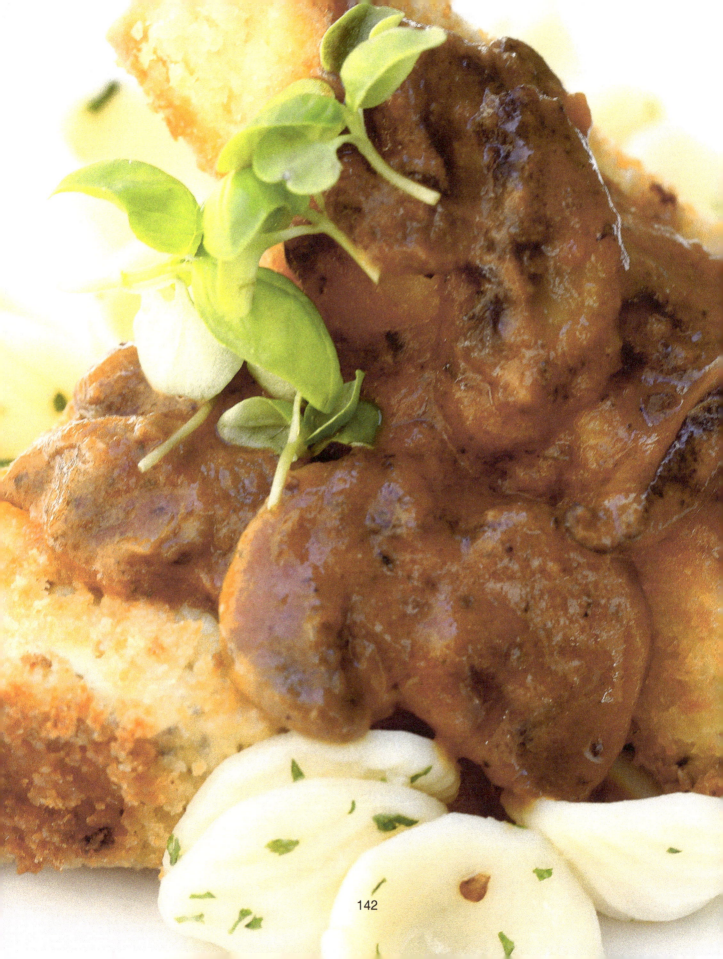

Tofu Marsala

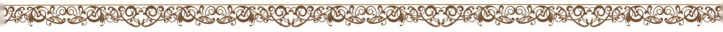

Ingredients:

- 1 cup of Italian Bread Crumbs
- ¼ teaspoon salt
- ¼ teaspoon freshly ground pepper
- 1 14-ounce block extra-firm tofu (cut crosswise into eight ½-inch-thick slices)
- 4 tablespoons extra-virgin olive oil, divided
- 2 large shallots, minced
- 1 teaspoon dried thyme
- 10 ounces sliced cremini mushrooms
- ½ cup dry Marsala wine
- 1 cup vegetable broth
- 1 tablespoon tomato paste

Instructions:

Pre heat oven to 300 degrees.

Heat 2 tablespoons oil in a large nonstick skillet over medium-high heat. Dredge 4 tofu slices in the bread crumbs, add them to the pan, and cook until crispy and golden, about 3 minutes per side. Place the tofu on a baking sheet, and transfer to the oven to keep warm. Repeat with another tablespoon of oil and the remaining tofu, adjusting the heat if necessary to prevent scorching.

Add the remaining 1 tablespoon oil, shallots, and thyme to the pan. Reduce heat to medium and cook, stirring constantly, until the shallots are slightly soft and beginning to brown, 1 to 2 minutes. Add mushrooms and cook, stirring often, until tender and lightly browned, 3 to 5 minutes. Add salt and pepper.

Stir in marsala, tomato paste, and broth, and simmer until slightly reduced, about 4 minutes. Sauce should look glossy and thick. Spoon the sauce over the tofu, and serve hot with your favorite pasta. Orecchiette is pictured with our tofu marsala.

Yields 4 to 5 servings

Zucchini Tempura with Mushroom Pear Ragout

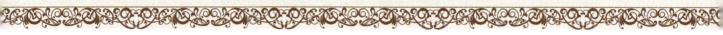

Ingredients:

6 large zucchini squash cut lengthwise

1 cup cake flour

½ teaspoon salt

½ teaspoon sugar

1 teaspoon baking powder

1 cup cold water

3 tablespoons vegetable oil

2 cups oil for frying

mushroom pear ragout (see recipe on page 131)

Instructions:

Combine cake flour, salt, sugar, and baking powder. Slowly add the oil and water until smooth and creamy. Chill for at least 30 minutes.

Heat 3 cups of vegetable oil in a wok or large frying pan over high heat. Dip the vegetables in the batter, and drop into the oil. Allow to cook for about 3 minutes, until crisp and lightly golden brown. Drain on paper towels.

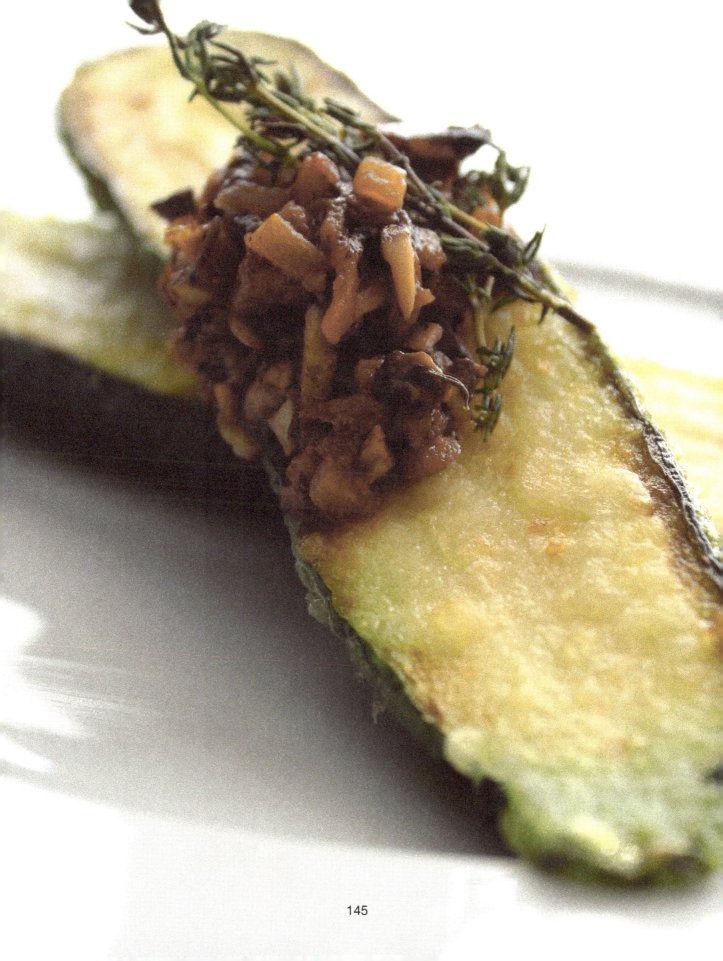

Gnocchi with Tempeh and Eggplant Bolognese

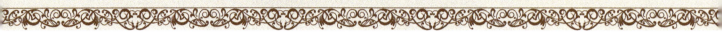

Ingredients:

- 1 block of tempeh
- 1 large eggplants
- 16 ounces of marinara sauce
- 1 pound gnocchi pasta
- 4 large leaves of fresh basil
- 8 ounces asiago cheese
- 1 cup of tamari sauce
- 2 tablespoons extra virgin olive oil

Instructions:

Preheat the oven to 375 degrees.

Cut the tempeh in bite-sized pieces, and marinate for 30 minutes in tamari sauce, olive oil, and black pepper.

Cut eggplant in cubes, and add salt. Let stand for 30 minutes until the eggplant releases excess water. After 30 minutes, drain eggplant on paper towels.

Toss eggplant cubes in olive oil and black pepper, and place them on a baking sheet.

Place in preheated oven, and bake for 25 minutes, turning intermittently at about 12 minutes for each side. On another baking sheet, add the marinated tempeh to the oven while the eggplant is baking. Allow tempeh to cook for 25 minutes as well.

Wash the basil and chiffonade.

In a large pot, boil water and add salt. Add the gnocchi, and reduce heat to medium high. Cook for 3 to 5 minutes, or until gnocchi floats atop the water. When the tempeh and eggplant finished cooking, transfer them to a big pot, and add the tomato sauce, fresh basil, and asiago cheese. Salt and pepper to taste.

Yields 4 to 5 servings

Seitan Chicken, Eggplant, and Mushroom Curry

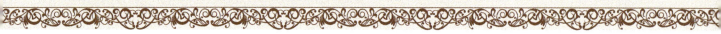

Ingredients:

- 2 pounds of seitan chicken cut into strips
- 1 medium eggplant
- 1 can of baby corn
- ½ pound of sugar snap peas
- 2 tablespoons of cooking oil
- 1 tablespoon of sesame seed oil
- 2 tablespoons red curry paste
- 12 ounces coconut milk
- 1 red bell pepper cut into strips
- 8 ounces fresh mushrooms (I used a wild mushroom mix)
- 2 scallions chopped

Instructions:

Preheat oven to 375 degrees.

Cut eggplant into cubes. Salt and let drain in a colander for 20 to 30 minutes. After the eggplant has rested in the salt bath for allotted time, rinse gently in cold water, and pat dry.

Toss the cubes in 2 tablespoons of olive oil, and place in a single layer on baking sheet. Place in preheated oven, and cook for 20 minutes until roasted.

Heat a skillet over medium-high heat. Once hot, add the cooking oil and red curry paste. Whisk for about 30 seconds. Pour in the coconut milk, and whisk to combine. When it comes to a simmer, add in the mushrooms, scallions, corn, snap peas, and red bell peppers. Continue cooking for 3 minutes. Add the seitan chicken strips to the curry, and cook for another 10 to 12 minutes, until the seitan is cooked through. Add the roasted eggplant to the curry mixture, and serve with rice.

Yields 4 to 5 servings

Chapter 6

Desserts

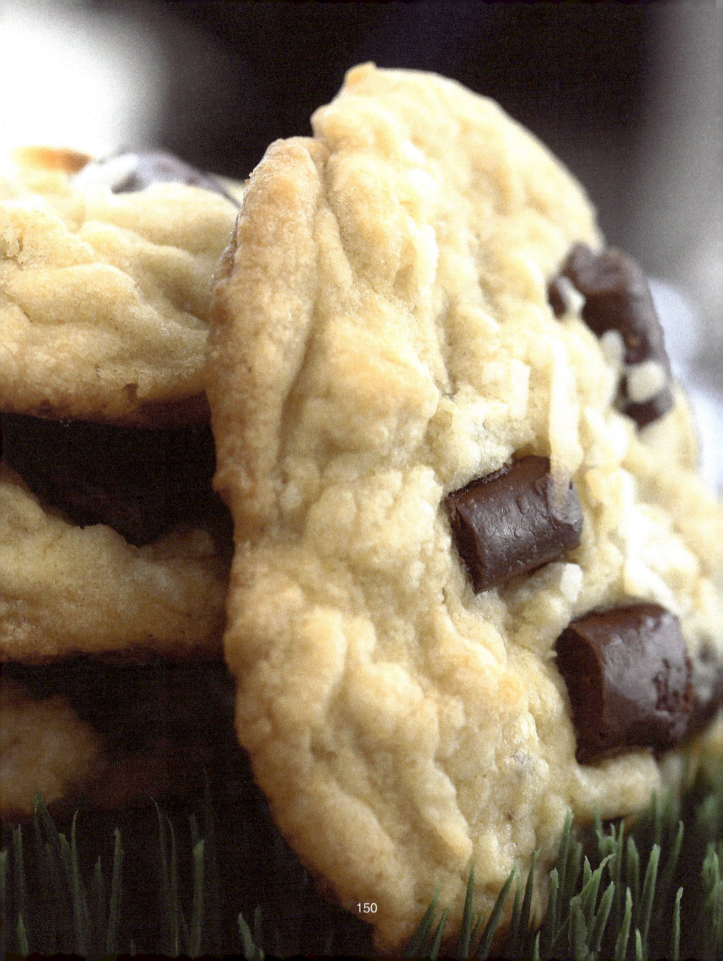

Chocolate Chunk Coconut Cookies

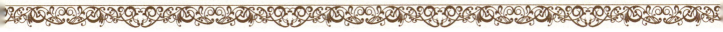

Ingredients:

- 2 ¼ cups all-purpose flour
- 1 teaspoon baking soda
- 1 teaspoon salt
- 1 cup butter, softened (2 sticks, ½ pounds)
- ¾ cups granulated sugar (white)
- ¾ cups packed brown sugar
- 1 teaspoon vanilla extract
- 3 teaspoons dry egg replacer plus 4 tablespoons water
- 2 cups vegan bittersweet chocolate chunks
- 1 cup shredded coconut

Instructions:

Combine flour, baking soda, and salt in small bowl. Using a hand mixer, beat the granulated sugar, butter, brown sugar, and vanilla in large mixer bowl. Mix the dry egg replacer with water, and add to the vegan butter mixture until the ingredients are mixed well. Mix in the flour mixture, and stir in chocolate chunks and coconut. Drop by rounded tablespoons onto ungreased baking sheets.

Bake in preheated 375-degree oven for 9 to 11 minutes or until golden brown. Let stand for 2 minutes; remove to wire racks to cool completely.

Makes 2 dozen cookies.

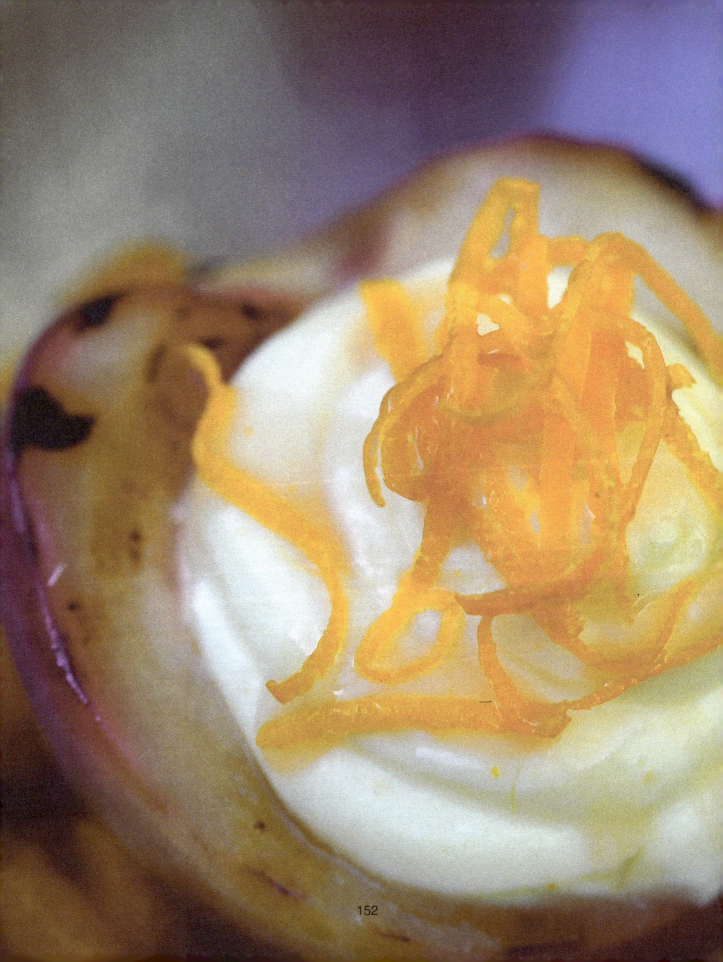

Grilled Macerated Peaches with Feta and Mascarpone Orange Cream

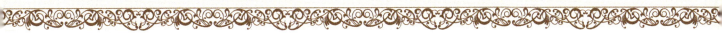

Ingredients:

1 pound white flesh peaches, cut into halves
½ cups sugar
¼ cups limoncello
1 tablespoon fresh grated ginger
¼ teaspoons ground nutmeg
¼ teaspoons cinnamon
orange zest curls for garnish

Instructions:

In a glass container, combine all the ingredients together. Allow the peaches to marinate overnight. Remove peach halves from the marinade liquid. Reserve the liquid for the glaze.

Preheat grill, and grill macerated peach halves on the cut side facedown. Grill for about 2 minutes on each side until the peaches have grill marks. Allow peaches to rest, and pipe the feta and mascarpone orange cream (*see recipe below) into the center of each peach half. Garnish with orange zest curls.

Yield 3 to 4 servings

Feta and Mascarpone Orange Cream

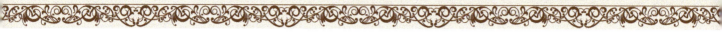

Ingredients:

- ½ cup feta cheese
- 1 cup mascarpone
- ¼ cup heavy whipping cream
- 1 cup confectioner's sugar
- 2 tablespoons of freshly squeezed orange juice
- ½ orange zest

Instructions:

In a mixing bowl, add crumbled feta, mascarpone, and orange juice. Using a hand mixer, mix the cheeses and orange just on a medium-speed setting until fluffy.

Gradually add the confectioner's sugar, and mix until the mixture is firm but has soft peaks. Add the heavy cream, and continue to mix until the mixture is spreadable about 2 to 3 minutes (do not overwhip as the cream will begin to break).

Gently fold in the orange zest, and serve with your favorite fruits or as a frosting for cupcakes.

Yield 3 to 4 servings

Mini Sticky Rice with Cardamom Coconut Milk and Mango Coulee

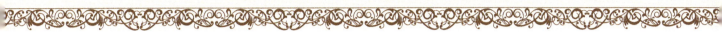

Ingredients:

1 cup Thai sweet rice

1 8-ounce can coconut milk

3 tablespoons raw sugar plus 2 tablespoons for coulee

1 pinch of cardamom powder

1 teaspoon kosher salt, divided

½ teaspoon cornstarch

2 ripe mangos, plus ¼ cup small dice

mango nectar for garnish

Instructions:

Soak 1 cup of dry sticky rice in water for about 2 to 4 hours. The longer the rice soaks, the softer it will be when it cooks.

Drain the rice, and rinse it thorough. Then pour about 1 cup of water into a saucepan, and place the rice in a steamer insert inside the saucepan. Cover tightly, and steam over low to medium heat for 30 to 40 minutes.

Open the can of coconut milk, and remove the thick cream on top.

Place the thicker coconut cream in a small bowl. You should have approximately ½ cup.

Pour the thinner, lighter coconut milk left in the can into a small saucepan. Stir in 2 tablespoons sugar and a pinch of cardamom powder. Warm over medium heat, stirring frequently for 5 minutes. Do not let the sauce boil.

By now, the rice is probably done soaking. The grains should be tender and shiny. Spoon the rice out into a bowl (it will be clumpy).

Slowly pour the warm coconut milk over the rice in the bowl, stirring frequently. You want the milk to coat the rice. Keep stirring, and stop pouring in coconut milk when it looks like the rice is saturated. Set the rice aside to finish absorbing the coconut milk, approximately 15 to 20 minutes.

While the rice is standing, make the coconut topping sauce. Rinse out the coconut milk saucepan, and pour in the coconut cream that you took off the top of the can. Stir in 1 tablespoon sugar. In a separate bowl, whisk together a few teaspoons of water and the cornstarch. Whisk this cornstarch slurry into the coconut cream, and cook over low heat for about 3 minutes, or until the mixture thickens considerably. Set aside.

Next placed the diced mango, nectar, and sugar in a pot over medium heat. Cook the mango mixture for about 10 to 12 minutes until the liquid reduces and the sugar dissolves. Remove from heat, and strain the mixture in a chinois. The liquid mixture should be syrupy but not thick. Cool the coulee.

To serve, place about ¼ cup cooked sticky rice into a ring mold. Using your forefinger, remove the rice from the molds, and place each round of sticky rice on individual plates.

Next, using a teaspoon, dot each plate with the mango coulee. Drizzle with the coconut topping sauce.

Garnish with a mint sprig and diced mango. Eat while still warm.

Yields 4 to 5 servings

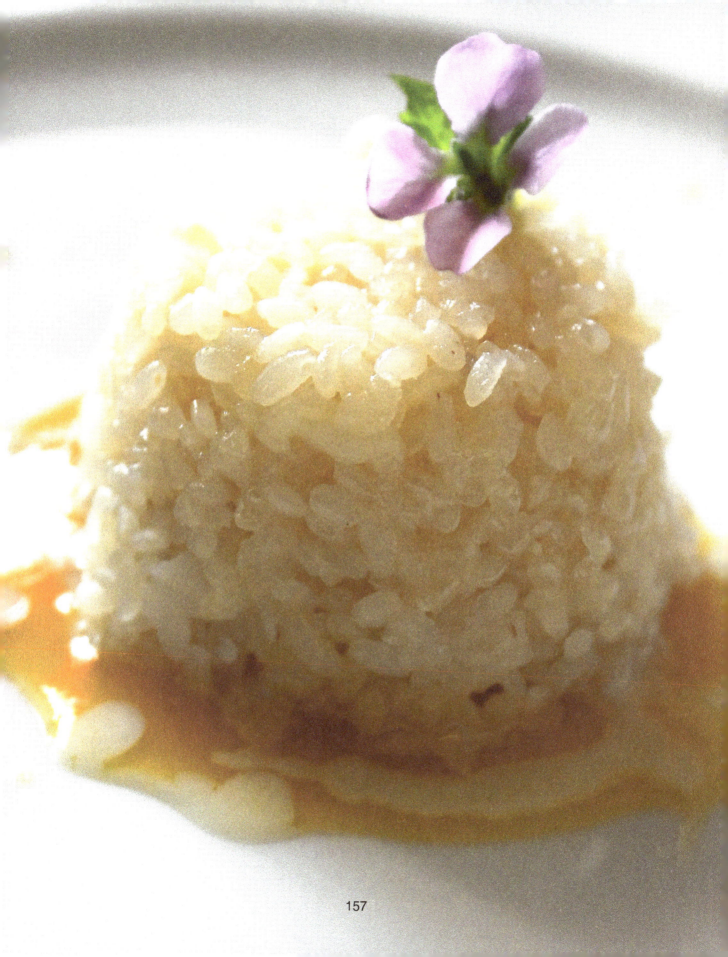

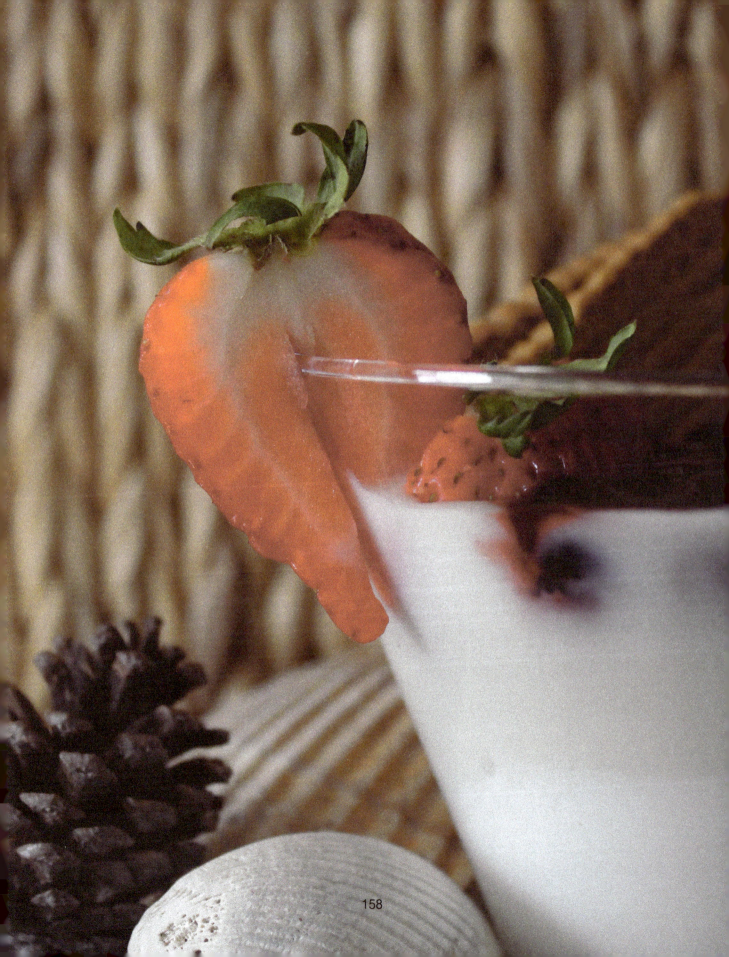

White Chocolate Coconut Crème Anglaise

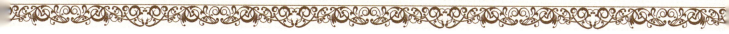

Ingredients:

½ cup white chocolate pieces

¼ cups sugar

3 tablespoons cornstarch

7 ounces coconut milk

1 cup almond milk

1 vanilla bean, scraped

Instructions:

Heat coconut milk and almond milk in a pot over medium heat. Do not allow milk to boil. Add the vanilla bean, and stir the milk mixture, making sure the milks do not scorch. After 5 minutes, remove vanilla bean, and scrape the beans from the hull. Add the vanilla beans back to the pot.

Sift together cornstarch, and add to the milk mixture. Continue to stir. Reduce heat to medium low.

Add the white chocolate pieces, and stir until the pieces have melted and the mixture has slightly thickened.

Serve at room temperature with ***Port Wine Fresh Berry Compote** (see recipe on page 162).

Yields 2 to 3 servings

Avocado Gelato

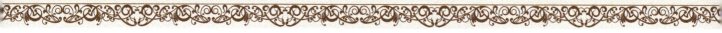

Ingredients:

- 3 ripe avocados
- 1 frozen banana
- 1 cup coconut cream (the thick cream that forms at the top of a can of full-fat coconut milk)
- ½ cup honey
- 2 tablespoon fresh lime juice
- 1 teaspoon pure vanilla extract
- ¼ teaspoon salt
- 4 Biscoff cookies (crumbled)

Instructions:

Remove the pits from the avocados. Remove the thick cream from the top of the coconut milk. Blend all ingredients together in a blender on high speed.

Turn off blender, and remove the avocado mixture. Place the creamed ingredients into an ice cream maker, and follow the directions to freeze the gelato. Churn the gelato for approximately 15 to 17 minutes until it has come to a hardened-but-still-creamy texture.

Serve your gelato over the crumbled Biscoff cookies.

Yields 3 to 4 servings

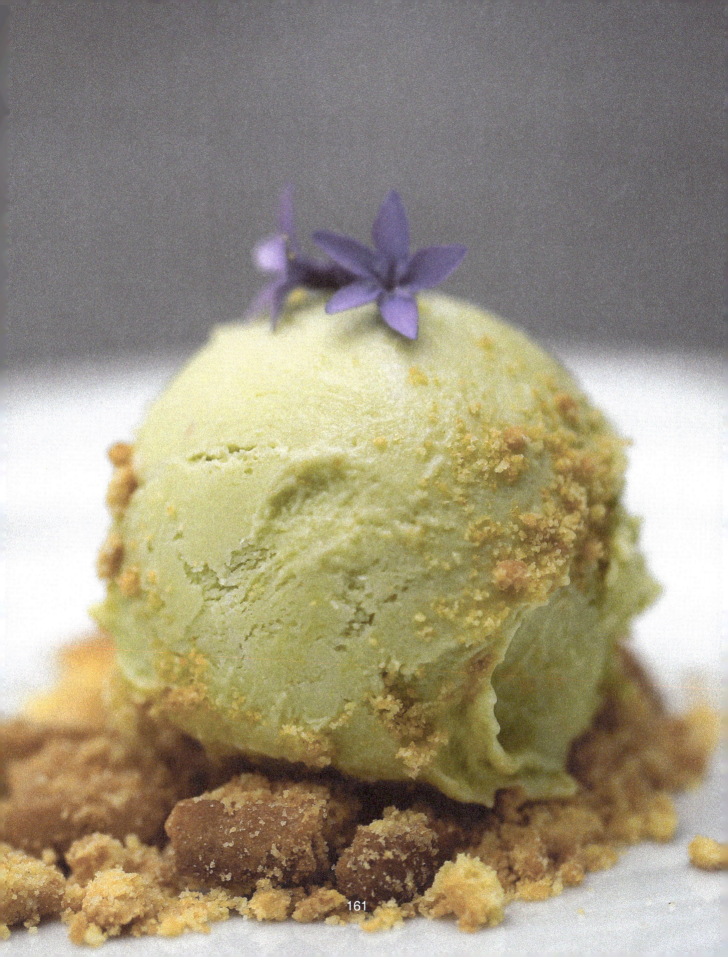

Port Wine Fresh Berry Compote

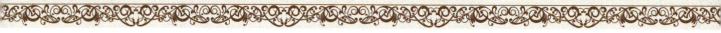

Ingredients:

- ½ cup blueberries
- ½ cup strawberries, stems removed and diced
- ½ cup raspberries
- ½ tablespoons pomegranate juice
- 1 teaspoon lime juice
- ¼ cup of port wine
- ½ cup pure cane sugar

Instructions:

Add berries, pomegranate juice, lime juice, sugar and port wine to a sauce pot.

Bring to a simmer and cook, stirring occasionally until the berries thicken the liquid but maintain their textures, approximately 7 minutes.

Yields 2 to 3 servings

Chapter 7

Breakfast

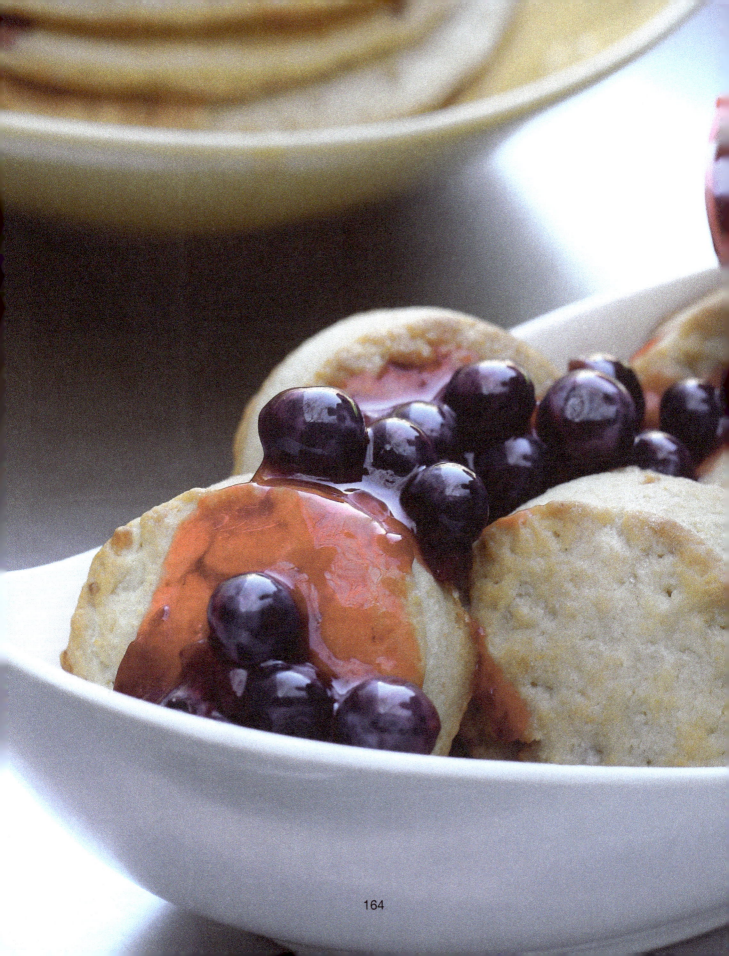

Blue Cheese Buttermilk Scones with Blueberry and Strawberry Compote

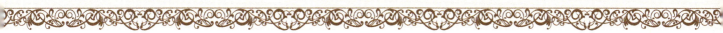

Ingredients:

- 3 cups all-purpose flour
- ½ cups white sugar
- 5 teaspoons baking powder
- ½ teaspoon salt
- 1-pound unsalted butter
- 1 cup of buttermilk
- 1 cup blue cheese
- 1 ½ tablespoon egg replacer plus 2 tablespoons of water
- blueberry strawberry compote (see recipe below)

Instructions:

Preheat oven to 400 degrees. Lightly grease a baking sheet.

In a large bowl, combine flour, sugar, baking powder, and salt. Cut in butter. Mix the egg replacer with the water, and add to the buttermilk in a small bowl. Add the flour mixture and blue cheese, and stir the combined ingredients until moistened.

Turn dough out onto a lightly floured surface, and knead briefly. Roll dough out into a half-inch-thick round. Using a biscuit cutter, cut into 8 rounds, and place on the prepared baking sheet.

Bake for 15 minutes in the preheated oven, or until golden brown. Serve each scone with a spoonful of blueberry and strawberry compote.

Yields 8 scones

Blueberry and Strawberry Compote

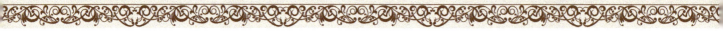

Ingredients:

- 1 cup port wine
- ¼ cup sugar
- 1 cinnamon stick
- 4 cups sliced strawberries
- 1 cup blueberries

Instructions:

Combine port wine, sugar, and cinnamon stick in a small nonstick saucepan; bring to a boil. Reduce heat; simmer, uncovered, 20 minutes or until liquid is reduced to ½ cup.

Drain wine mixture in a colander over a large bowl; discard solids. Add berries; toss to coat. Serve warm or chill up to 2 hours.

Yields 2 to 3 servings

Chia and Hemp Seed Porridge

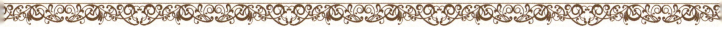

Ingredients:

- 2 cups coconut milk, unsweetened
- 1 teaspoon kosher sea salt
- ½ cups hemp seed, freshly ground
- ½ cups chia seed

Instructions:

Bring coconut milk to just below a simmer.

Whisk in sea salt and hemp seed. Bring mixture to a boil, and simmer for 5 minutes.

Remove from heat, and whisk in chia seeds.

Let the mixture thicken for 10 minutes, and serve porridge with desired toppings.

Yields 3 to 4 servings

Maple Tempeh Bacon with Creamy Gorgonzola Grits

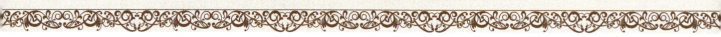

Ingredients:

See recipe for maple tempeh bacon on page 172.

Grits

1 tablespoon olive oil
1 cup grits
4 cups water
½ cup heavy cream
½ cup gorgonzola cheese, crumbled
salt and white pepper to taste
finely chopped chives for garnish

Instructions:

Heat about 1 tablespoon oil in a skillet, and add the tempeh pieces in a single layer. Cook a few minute on each side until browned.

To make the grits, bring the water to a boil, and stir in the grits, mixing well to get rid of any lumps. Bring to a boil, then turn down and simmer until thickened, stirring frequently for about 10 minutes. Add the heavy cream, gorgonzola cheese, and a pinch of salt and white pepper. Continue simmering until soft and thickened, another 15 minutes or so.

To serve, put the grits in a bowl and top with chopped tempeh, gorgonzola, and chives.

Yields 3 to 4 servings

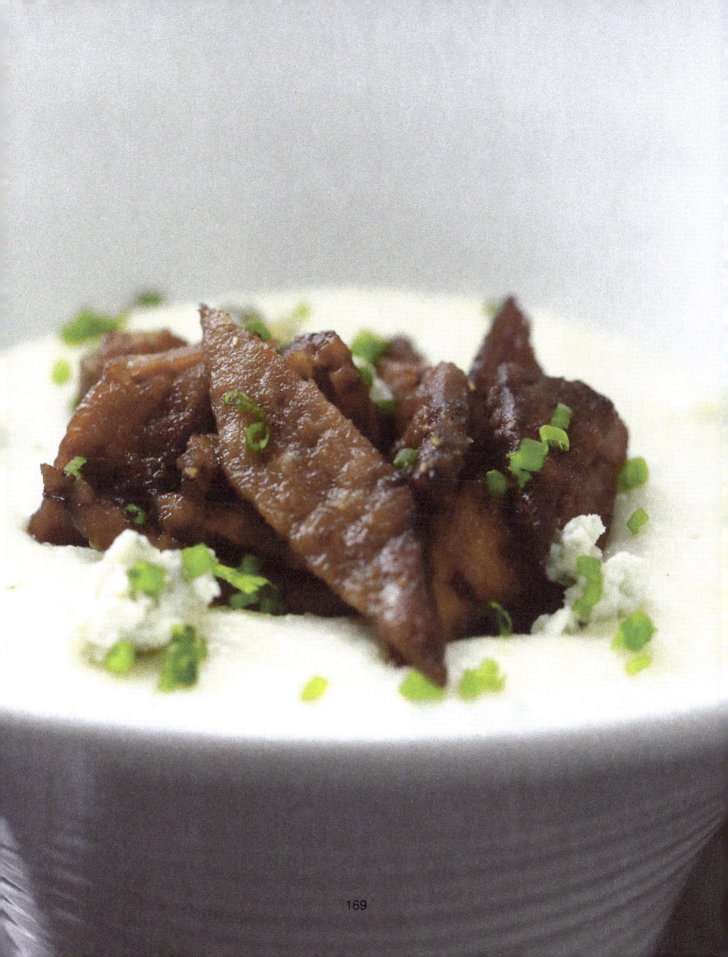

Banana Coconut Pancake Stack with Cashew Butter

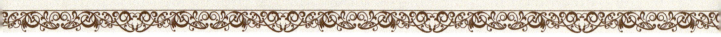

Ingredients:

Pancake Batter:

- 3 each overripe bananas
- 1 teaspoon vanilla extract
- 1 teaspoon kosher sea salt
- 3 tablespoons ground flax seed
- 2 cups coconut milk, unsweetened
- ½ cups coconut flour
- ¼ cups tapioca flour
- 2 tablespoons coconut oil, melted
- 2 teaspoons cinnamon, ground
- 1 tablespoon baking powder

Yields 3 to 4 servings

Cashew Butter

Ingredients:

- 6 ounces cashew butter, fresh ground
- 3 ounces agave nectar
- 1 teaspoon kosher sea salt

Instructions:

Preheat a nonstick griddle to 350°F.

Combine first set of ingredients in a blender, and puree until velvety smooth. Allow to rest for 5 minutes, Puree one more time. Ladle 3ounce of the batter onto the griddle, and cook for 4–5 minutes, until golden brown and slightly dry around edges.

Flip each pancake, and cook for an additional 3 to 4 minutes until fluffy and cooked through.

Remove from the griddle, and reserve to the side. Continue process with remaining batter.

Meanwhile, combine cashew butter, agave nectar, and sea salt.

As pancakes come off of the griddle, spread an even layer of cashew butter on the pancakes.

Yields 3 to 4 servings

Maple Tempeh Bacon

Ingredients:

- 8 ounces tempeh
- 1–2 tablespoons maple syrup
- 1 tablespoon olive oil
- ½ teaspoons cumin
- a dash cayenne
- 1 teaspoon liquid smoke
- 1 teaspoon soy sauce
- ½ teaspoons coarse black pepper and sea salt
- 2 teaspoons olive oil for cooking tempeh

Instructions:

Thinly slice tempeh as thin as you can without it falling apart.

Next, combine all ingredients in a shallow dish, and soak tempeh in marinade for 1–2 minutes.

Turn sauté pan on high; add 1–2 teaspoons olive oil. Lay the tempeh flat on skillet, one layer only. Drizzle a bit of excess marinade onto skillet; it should be sizzling a lot now.

Cook for 1 minute, then flip. Cook for another minute on the other side or until both sides are crisp and browned.

Place cooked tempeh on parchment paper to cool, and sprinkle with black pepper and sea salt to taste.

Note: For a crisper tempeh bacon, do not pour excess marinade in skillet, and allow all liquid to steam off pan while cooking.

Yields 3 to 4 servings

Chickpea Egg Scramble

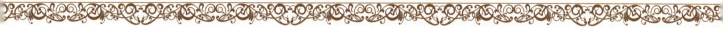

Ingredients:

¾ cups chickpea flour

¾ cups filtered water

1 tablespoon red miso paste

1 teaspoon white pepper, ground

1 teaspoon kosher sea salt (more if desired)

1 each onion, small dice

1 each bell pepper, small dice

1 each carrot, grated

1 each zucchini, grated

2 each garlic clove, minced

4 tablespoons coconut oil

1 tablespoon organic extra virgin olive oil (unfiltered preferred)

Instructions:

Using a whisk, combine chickpea flour, water, miso, pepper, and salt. Set aside to rest.

In a cast iron skillet, heat coconut oil over medium-low heat and add onion, bell pepper, carrot, and zucchini. Sauté until lightly caramelized (this will take approximately 15 minutes). Add garlic clove, and cook for an additional 2 minutes. Add chickpea batter to vegetable, stir to combine, then let "set up" for approximately 5 minutes. Stir to redistribute batter, then let remaining batter set up.

Serve with a fresh drizzle of organic olive oil, and more salt and pepper if desired.

Yields 4 to 5 servings

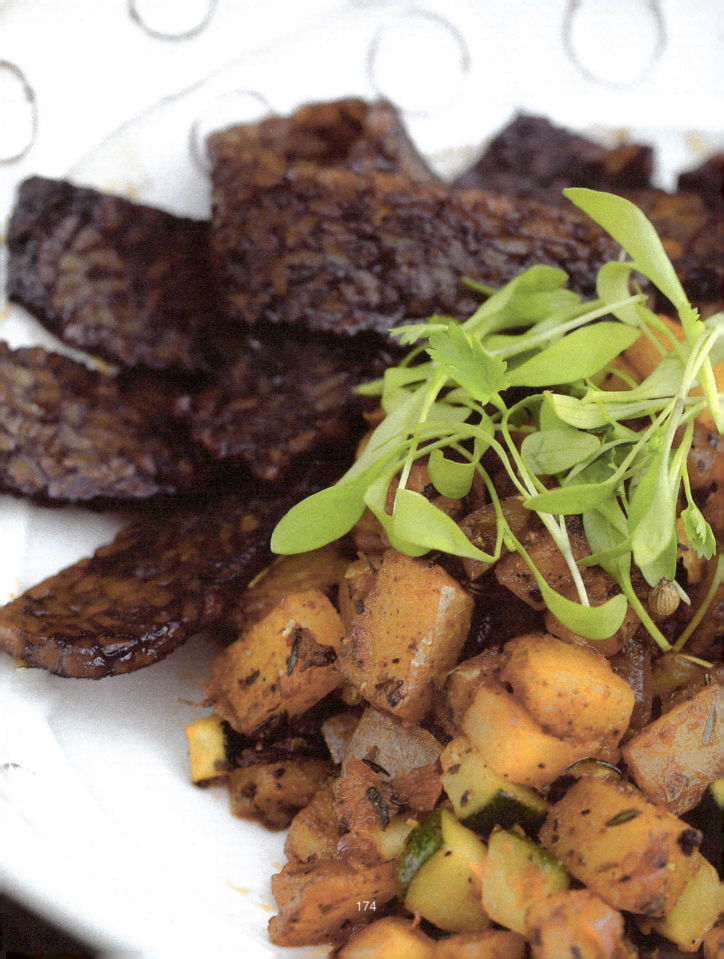

Vegan Potato and Zucchini Hash with Blackened Cajun Tempeh

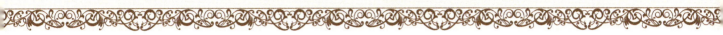

Ingredients:

- 1 tablespoon canola oil
- 1 cup onions (chopped)
- 1 cup green pepper (chopped)
- 1 cup diced potatoes
- 1 medium zucchini diced
- 2 teaspoons paprika
- ½ teaspoons garlic powder
- ½ teaspoons onion powder
- 1 pinch cayenne pepper
- blackened cajun tempeh (see recipe below)

Instructions:

Add oil to skillet, and heat over medium-high heat. Add onions, green bell pepper, and potatoes, and sauté for 5 to 7 minutes or until beginning to brown. Add diced zucchini, and continue to cook.

Sprinkle with paprika, garlic powder, onion powder, and cayenne pepper. Sauté 7 to 8 minutes, or until potatoes are browned and tender.

Yields 4 to 5 servings

Blackened Cajun Tempeh Bacon

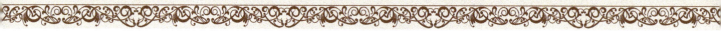

Ingredients:

tempeh strips, cut thin on a mandolin

½ teaspoon Cajun spice

½ teaspoon tamari

1 teaspoon ginger garlic paste

¼ teaspoon red chili powder or Cayenne pepper

¼ teaspoon black pepper or to taste

2 tablespoons canola oil

½ cup vegetable broth

Instructions:

Mix in all the ingredients, and pour the marinade over the tempeh strips. Allow the strips to marinade for at least 1 hour.

Heat canola oil in a skillet over medium heat, and add the strips to the pan. Make sure they are arranged individually and not overlapping one another.

Add the broth to the skillet just so they cover the tops of the strips. Cook the strips uncovered for approximately 10 minutes until the water has been absorbed.

Carefully turn the tempeh over, and cook for an additional 5 to 7 minutes. Continue to cook the strips in the same pan until the strips become blackened but not charred. Serve with the vegan potato and zucchini hash.

Yields 4 to 5 servings

Buckwheat Waffles with Gardein Chickenless Strips

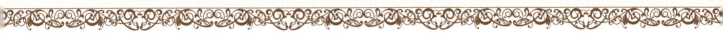

Ingredients:

- 1 cup buckwheat flour
- ½ cup almond flour
- 1 teaspoon baking powder
- ½ teaspoon kosher salt
- ½ teaspoon ground cinnamon
- 1 ½ tablespoon egg replacer plus 2 tablespoons of water
- 1 tablespoon coconut palm sugar
- 1 cup almond milk unsweetened
- ¼ cup coconut oil
- 1 package of Gardein chickenless strips

Instructions:

Mix the dry ingredients together in a bowl and set aside. Mix egg replacer with water until well mixed. Add to the sugar and milk and coconut oil, and mix.

Slowly whisk in the dry ingredients until moist. Let the batter stand in the bowl for 10 minutes before you use it.

For the chickenless strips, heat a sauté pan over medium high heat and add 2 tablespoons of canola oil. Lightly salt and pepper strips. Add strips to hot pan, and sauté for approximately 4 to 5 minutes. Remove from pan, and set aside.

Pour ½ cup at a time into an oiled waffle iron. Serve with Gardein chickenless strips.

Yields 4 to 5 servings

Vegetarian Strawberry Pancakes with Chocolate Almond Spread

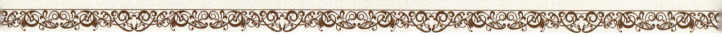

Ingredients:

2 cups cake flour

¼ cups cornstarch

2 tablespoons sugar

1 teaspoon salt

1 tablespoon baking powder

2 cups fresh strawberries, sliced

2 ½ cups coconut milk

2 tablespoons canola oil

chocolate almond spread (see recipe on page 181)

Instructions:

Mix dry ingredients. Add the coconut milk and canola oil. Blend the mixture until well mixed, but do not overmix.

Add sliced strawberries and mix until coated.

Add more flour or coconut as needed for the right consistency of the batter.

Pour enough batter on a medium-hot griddle, and flip. You see air bubbles in the batter, and the edges of the pancakes appear to be dry.

Spread pancakes with chocolate almond spread, and stack accordingly.

Yields 4 to 5 servings

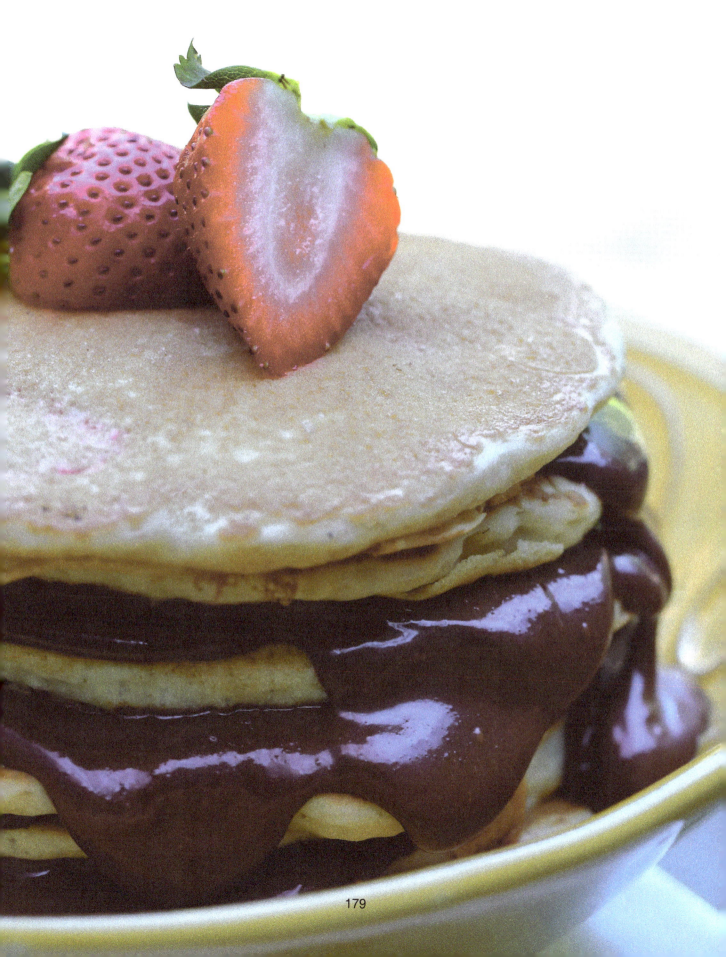

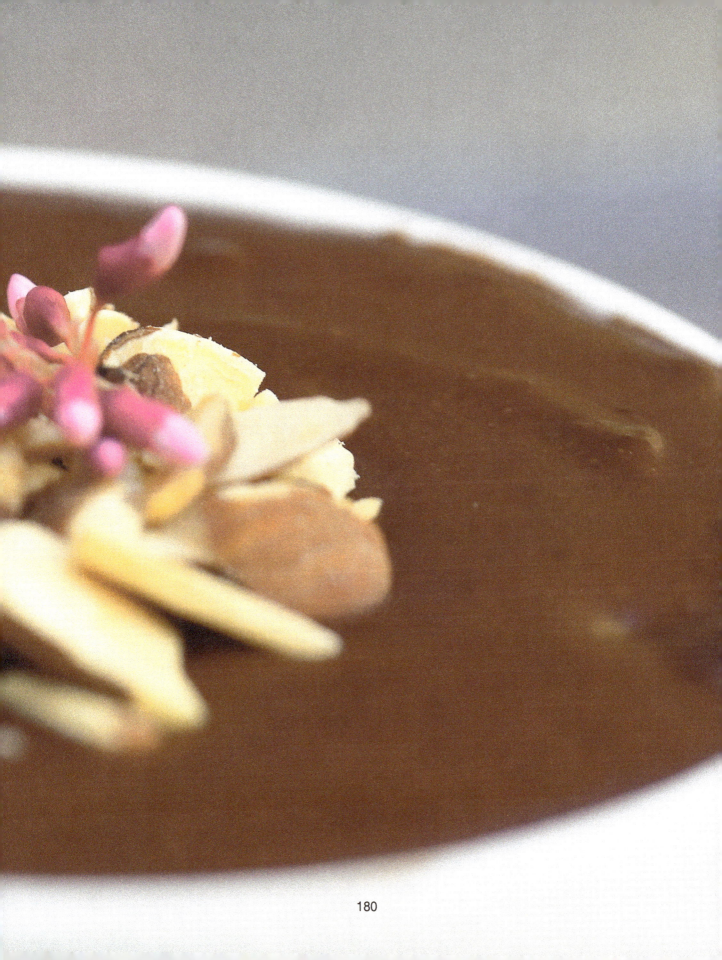

Chocolate Almond Spread

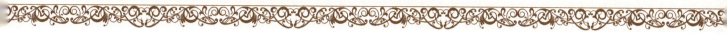

Ingredients:

- 1 cup toasted almonds
- 1 cup cocoa powder
- 3 ounces bittersweet chocolate (coarsely chopped)
- 4 ounces of coconut powder
- 2 tablespoons almond oil
- 3 tablespoons confectioner's sugar
- ½ teaspoons vanilla extract
- ¾ teaspoons kosher salt

Instructions:

Melt the chocolates in a double boiler until smooth.

In a blender or food processor, grind the almonds with the coconut powder until they break down into a fine powder. Add the oil, and process until it forms a smooth paste. Add the sugar, vanilla extract, and salt, and process until well incorporated.

Carefully add the melted chocolate; blend well.

Allow the chocolate spread to cool to room temperature; the spread will thicken up considerably upon cooling.

Yields 4 to 5 servings

Vegan, Gluten-Free, Dairy-Free Waffle Base

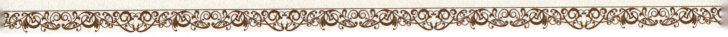

Ingredients:

- 5 cups coconut milk, unsweetened
- 1 cup applesauce, unsweetened
- 1 banana (as ripe as possible)
- 1 cup Pillsbury best gluten-free flour
- 1 cup coconut flour
- ½ cup tapioca flour
- ¼ cup garbanzo bean flour
- 1 tablespoon baking powder
- 2 teaspoons kosher salt
- 1 tablespoon vanilla bean extract (optional, see note)

Instructions:

Combine the first set of ingredients in a blender, and puree until smooth. Add remaining ingredients and pulse until incorporated and uniform. Allow batter to rest for 5 minutes for the liquid to be absorbed.

Portion onto a preheated and oiled waffle iron, and cook until golden brown and crisp.

Note: vanilla extract should only be used in sweet waffles; omit if savory waffles are being made.

Variations/enhancements:

Blueberry waffles with lemon ricotta and maple syrup

Peanut butter chip waffles with sliced banana and sweetened coconut whip

Diced apple waffles with salted caramel and pecans

Caramelized-shallots waffles with chikin, maple syrup, and hot sauce

Strawberry waffles with orange marmalade and sweetened coconut whipped cream

Smoked gouda waffle with mushroom and pearl onion ragu

Sweet potato cheddar waffle with maple grilled tofu, crispy onions, molasses

Yields 4 to 5 servings

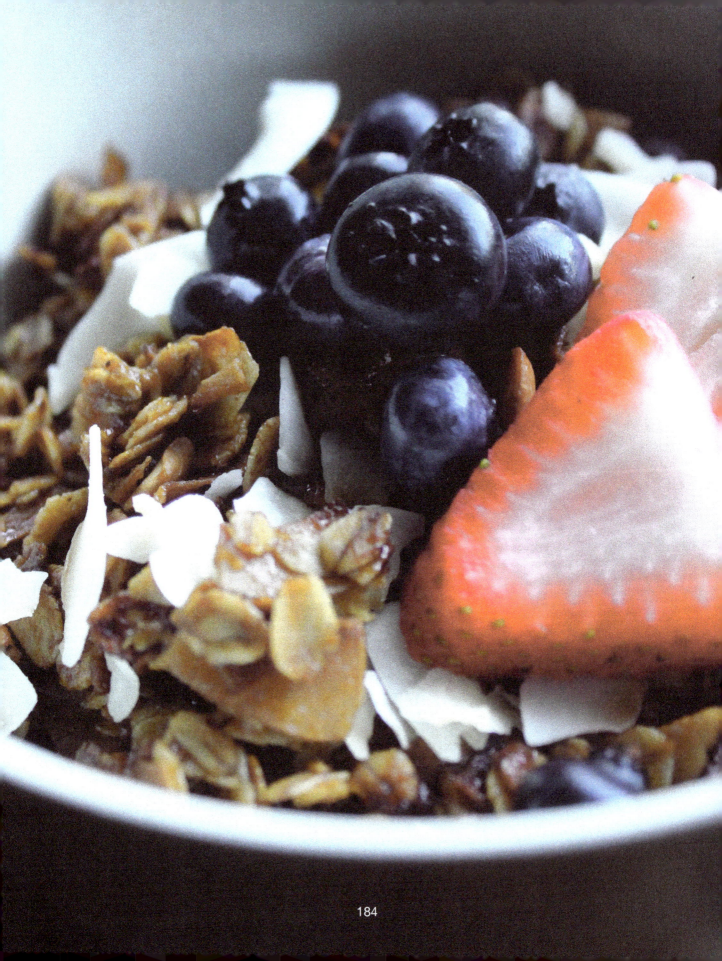

Good Morning Granola (Gluten-Free, Low Sugar, High Protein)

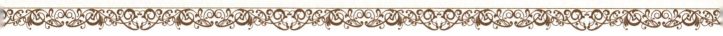

Ingredients:

4 cups rolled oats
4 cups unsweetened coconut
1 cup almonds, sliced
½ cup chia seed
½ cup flaxseed
3 cups textured vegetable protein
3 tablespoons nutritional yeast
1 tablespoon cinnamon
½ teaspoon cayenne pepper
½ teaspoon ground ginger
1 teaspoon kosher sea salt
½ cup maple syrup grade b
½ cup agave nectar
1 cup filtered water

Instructions:

Preheat convection oven to 350 conventional.

Prepare a half-size sheet pan lined with parchment. Spray pan with nonstick flavorless spray. Pack granola on the sheet pan, ensuring even thickness.

Bake 350 for 45 minutes. Then flip over the granola and return to sheet pan, keeping pieces as whole as possible.

Drop oven to 200 degrees, and dry out granola until desired texture is reached. (Chewy granola will take 30 minutes, and crunch granola will take up to 2 hours.) Cool and pack into an airtight container.

Yields 4 to 5 servings

Cheesy Tofu Scramble

Ingredients:

- 2 teaspoons earth balance buttery spread
- 1 container extra firm tofu, pressed and drained
- 1 tablespoon agave
- 2 teaspoons light miso paste
- 2 tablespoons fresh lemon juice
- ¼ teaspoon sea salt, plus to taste
- ¼ teaspoon finely ground black pepper, plus to taste
- ¼ teaspoon turmeric powder
- ¼ teaspoon garlic powder
- ½ bunch fresh chives, finely chopped
- ¼ cup daiya dairy-free smoked gouda shredded cheese

Instructions:

Heat a skillet over a medium heat, and add buttery spread.

Crumble tofu with your hands into a mixing bowl, and transfer to skillet. Add agave and lemon juice, and stir to incorporate.

Add sea salt, black pepper, turmeric, and garlic powder, and stir. Then add miso paste and stir to tofu scramble mixture. Cook for about 3–5 minutes, or until golden.

Add daiya shredded smoked gouda, and stir well for about 30 seconds to melt cheese and then remove from heat.

When serving, garnish with chives, and season to taste with additional sea salt and pepper.

Yields 4 to 5 servings

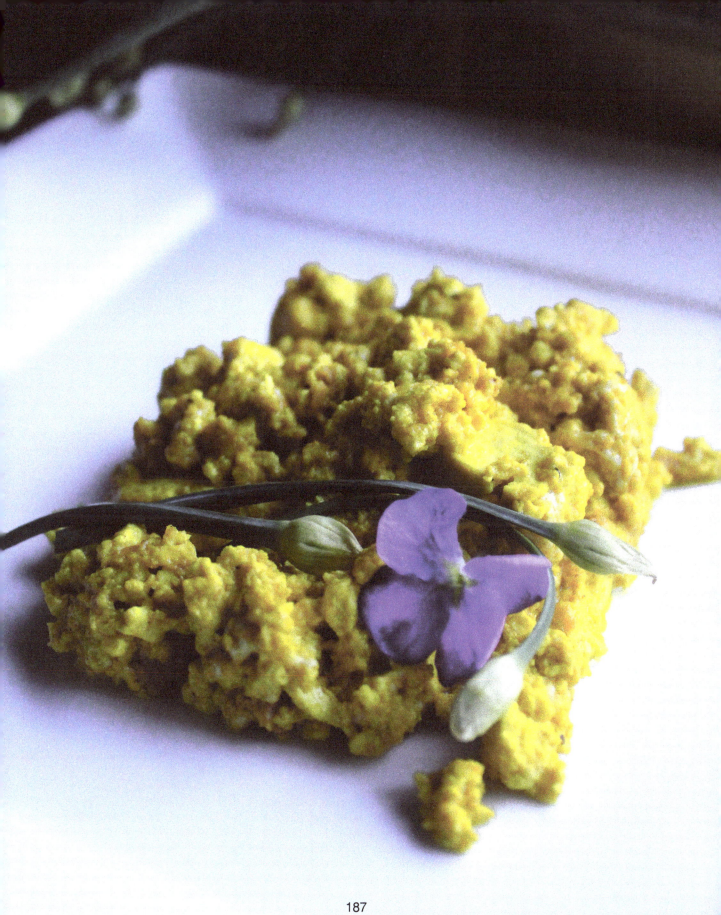

Chapter 8

Breads

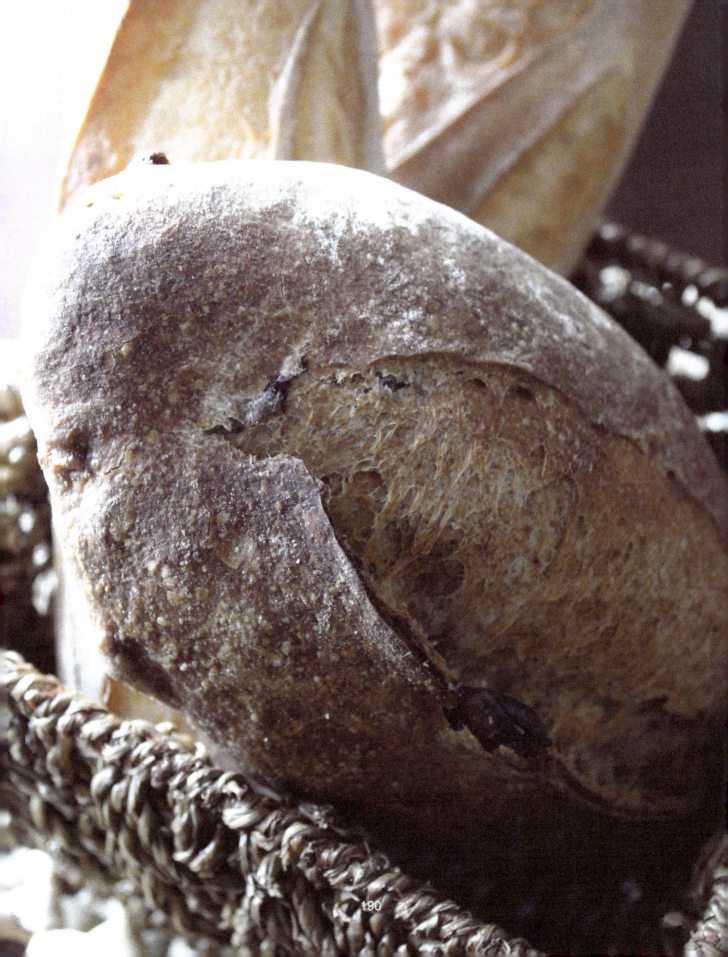

Whole Wheat Baguette

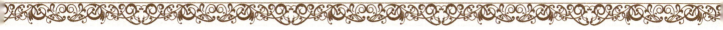

Ingredients:

1 ½ cups warm water
1 tablespoon instant yeast
2 cups whole wheat flour
2 cups white bread flour
1 tablespoon salt

Instructions:

Dissolve yeast in warm water (water should be at 90 degrees).

Fit your stand mixer with a bread paddle. Add the water to the bowl of the mixer. Add the flours and salt, and mix on low speed for about 3 minutes. Turn the mixer to a medium-speed setting, and mix for additional 2 minutes.

Remove the dough from the bowl, and place in well-oiled bowl. Cover for 1 hour or until the dough has doubled in size. Once the dough has risen, turn out onto lightly floured surface, and shape dough into a flattened oval.

Fold bottom third of dough over the middle, and press into dough. Then fold top third of dough to the bottom, and pinch to seal. Roll dough out until the crease is sealed and baguette has reached the desired length.

Dust baguette with flour and cover with towel. Let sit for one hour, or until baguette has risen.

Preheat oven to 425 degrees, and place a shallow pan of water on the bottom rack of the oven. Using a pastry brush, brush water along the top of the baguette. Using a very sharp knife, make three shallow slices along the length of the dough.

Place the baguette on a nonstick baking sheet on the rack above the rack with the shallow pan of water. Bake for 25 minutes, or until the baguette has a crispy crust and a deep, golden brown color.

Yields 1 baguette

Chocolate Banana Bread

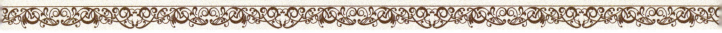

Ingredients:

- 2 cups all-purpose flour
- ¾ cups pure cane sugar
- ½ cup dark brown sugar, packed
- 1 ¼ cup bittersweet chocolate chunks
- ¾ teaspoons baking soda
- ¾ teaspoons salt
- ¾ teaspoons cinnamon
- ½ cup plain almond milk
- 1 teaspoon apple cider vinegar
- 2 cups mashed ripe bananas
- ¼ cup safflower oil
- 2 tablespoons agave
- 1 teaspoon pure vanilla extract

Instructions:

Preheat the oven to 350 F.

Lightly oil a 9×5 loaf pan and set aside.

In a medium-size mixing bowl, sift together the flour, sugars, baking soda, salt, and cinnamon.

In another larger mixing bowl, whisk together the almond milk and cider vinegar, and let rest for 2 minutes. Add the mashed banana, safflower oil, agave, and vanilla extract, whisking until well combined. Add the dry ingredients to the wet ingredients, and mix well until the ingredients are combined.

Fold in the chocolate chunks, and pour the batter into the prepared loaf pan. Bake for about 1 hour, or until a toothpick inserted into the center comes out clean. Allow the bread to cool on a wire cooling rack for 20 minutes before serving. Serve warm or at room temperature.

Yields 1 loaf

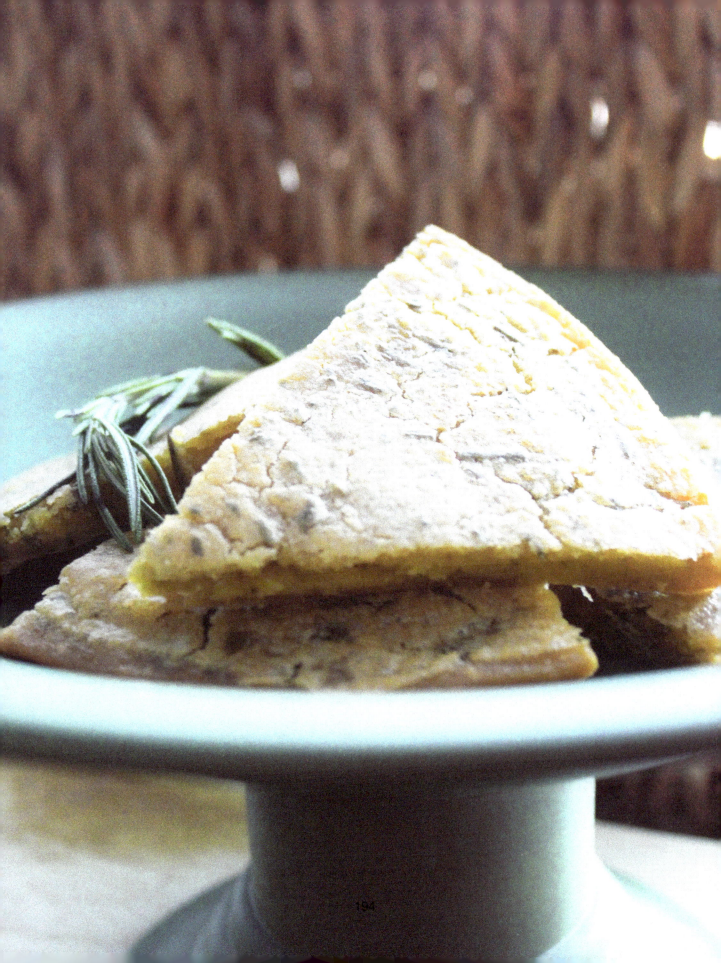

Farinata

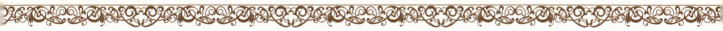

Ingredients:

½ pounds finely ground chickpea flour

1 teaspoon kosher salt

3 cups water

¼ cups extra-virgin olive oil

freshly ground black pepper

1 sprig of rosemary leaves, picked

Instructions:

Preheat oven to 550 degrees.

In a mixing bowl, combine chickpea flour and salt. Gradually add water, whisking constantly, until a smooth and a thin batter forms. Let the batter rest for 30 minutes, and then skim off any froth that has formed on the top of the batter.

Pour olive oil into seasoned large cast iron skillet, coating the bottom of the skillet. Stir batter to mix well, then pour into skillet. Stir gently to swirl oil on top of batter.

Season all over with black pepper, and sprinkle with rosemary leaves.

Turn on broiler, place the skillet into the oven, and cook until farinata has set and the edges are browned all over approximately 10 minutes.

Drizzle with a little extra virgin olive oil, and serve warm or at room temperature.

Yield 6 to 8 slices

Pizza Dough

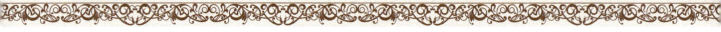

Ingredients:

- 2 teaspoons active dry yeast or instant yeast
- 1 ¼ cup lukewarm water
- 2 tablespoons olive oil
- 3 cups King Arthur unbleached all-purpose flour
- 1 ¼ teaspoon salt
- 2 teaspoons active dry yeast or instant yeast
- 7 to 9 ounces lukewarm water*
- ⅞ ounce olive oil
- 12 ¾ ounces King Arthur Unbleached All-Purpose Flour
- 1 ¼ teaspoons salt
- *Use the lesser amount in summer (or in a humid environment), the greater amount in winter (or in a dry climate), and somewhere in between the rest of the year, or if your house is climate controlled.

Instructions:

If you're using active dry yeast, dissolve it with a pinch of sugar in 2 tablespoons of the lukewarm water. Let the yeast and water sit at room temperature for 15 minutes, until the mixture has bubbled and expanded. If you're using instant yeast, you can skip this step.

Combine the dissolved yeast (or the instant yeast) with the remainder of the ingredients. Mix and knead everything together—by hand, mixer, or bread machine set on the dough cycle—till you've made a soft, smooth dough. If you're kneading in a stand mixer, it should take 4 to 5 minutes at second speed, and the dough should barely clean the sides of the bowl, perhaps sticking a bit at the bottom. Don't overknead the dough; it should hold together but can still look fairly rough on the surface.

To make pizza now: Place the dough in a lightly greased bowl, cover the bowl, and allow it to rise till it's very puffy. This will take about an hour using instant yeast, or 90 minutes using active dry. If it takes longer, that's okay; just give it some extra time.

To make pizza later: Allow the dough to rise, covered, for 45 minutes at room temperature. Refrigerate the dough for 4 hours (or for up to 24 hours); it will rise slowly as it chills. This step allows you more schedule flexibility; it also develops the crust's flavor. About 2 to 3 hours before you want to serve pizza, remove the dough from the refrigerator.

Yields 1 Pizza Pie

Recipe from King Arthur flour.

"You existed to teach me, and I still have many lessons to learn."

(Chef Bev)

Index

Salad Dressings and Marinades

Veganaise	7
Buttermilk Yogurt Dressing	8
Basic Vinaigrette	9
Balsamic Vinaigrette	10
Champagne Vinaigrette	11
Dijon Vinaigrette	12
Herb Oil Marinade	13
Barbecue Sauce	14
Tamari Ginger Marinade	16
Chermoula	17
Moroccan Spice Mix	19

Sauces, Dips, and Stocks

Chef Bev's Chimichurri	23
Tomato Glaze	24
Mojo Sauce	25
Blond Vegetable Stock	26
Brown Vegetable Stock	27
White Wine Sauce	28
Chef Bev's Romesco Sauce	29
Alfredo Sauce	30
Cucumber Cilantro Sauce	31
Tomato Sauce	32
Lemon Dill Sauce	33
Sun-Dried Tomato and Roasted Garlic Sauce	34
Roasted Eggplant with Gorgonzola Cheese Pasta Sauce	35
Grilled Artichoke Marinara Parmigiano	36
Classic Marinara Sauce	39
Kale and Tarragon Pesto	41

Appetizers

Muhammara	45
Baba Ghanouj	47
Hummus	49
Chef Bev's Labneh	51
Labneh Crostini with Tofurkey Italian Sausage, Dried Apricots, and Thyme	53
Sicilian Caponata	54
Mini Black Bean Cakes	56

Soups, Salads, and Sides

Papaya Gazpacho	61
Grilled Asparagus with Herb Oil Marinade	65
Tomato Concasse Caprese with Balsamic Pearls and Microgreens	67
*Balsamic Pearls	68

Jicama and Pomelo Salad	69
Thai Kale Salad	70
Watermelon, Feta, and Mint Caprese	72
Coconut Cauliflower Rice	73
Cauliflower Veloute with Wild Mushrooms and Balsamic Pearls	74
Ful Mudammas	76
Savory Bread Pudding with Mushrooms	79
Quinoa Salad with Cranberries and Spinach	81
Papa al Pomodoro (Tuscan Bread Soup)	82
Chilled Avocado and Coconut Soup with Macerated Grapes	85
Glazed Brussels Sprouts	86
Superfood Bowl with Fresh Kale, Brussels Sprouts, Quinoa, and Hempseeds with Green Goddess Dressing	87
Vegan Causa (Peruvian Mashed Potato Salad)	89
Mango and Avocado Ceviche	93

Main Dishes

Risotto with Asparagus and Wild Mushrooms	97
Chickenless Mexican Stew	99
Curried Lentil Stew	100
Creamy Saffron Risotto with Sautéed Brussels Sprouts and Chanterelles	102
Chef Bev's Mushroom, Zucchini, and Yellow Squash Veggie Burgers	105
Roasted Cauliflower Meuniere	107
General Tzo's Cauliflower	109
Chickenless Milano	111
Kimchi Pancakes	113
Braised Eggplant with Tofu in Garlic Sauce	114
Ratatouille	117
Moroccan Beefless Kebabs with Chermoula	119
Gruyere Polenta Cakes with Sun-Dried Tomato Caper Quenelles and Alfredo Sauce	121
Dynamite Tofu	123
Butter Curry Seitan	125
Ground Nut Stew	127
Cauliflower Piccata	129
Mushroom Pear Ragout	131
Wild Mushroom Pizza with Alfredo Sauce	133
Roasted Eggplant Masala (Baingan Bharta)	135
Easy Feijoada	139
Vegan Bolognese	140
Tofu Marsala	143
Zucchini Tempura with Mushroom Pear Ragout	144
Gnocchi with Tempeh and Eggplant Bolognese	146
Seitan Chicken, Eggplant, and Mushroom Curry	148

Desserts

Chocolate Chunk Coconut Cookies	151
Grilled Macerated Peaches with Feta and Mascarpone Orange Cream	153

Feta and Mascarpone Orange Cream	154
Mini Sticky Rice with Cardamom Coconut Milk and Mango Coulee	155
White Chocolate Coconut Crème Anglaise	159
Avocado Gelato	160
Port Wine Fresh Berry Compote	162

Breakfast

Blue Cheese Buttermilk Scones with Blueberry and Strawberry Compote	165
Blueberry and Strawberry Compote	166
Chia and Hemp Seed Porridge	167
Maple Tempeh Bacon with Creamy Gorgonzola Grits	168
Banana Coconut Pancake Stack with Cashew Butter	170
Maple Tempeh Bacon	172
Chickpea Egg Scramble	173
Vegan Potato and Zucchini Hash with Blackened Cajun Tempeh	175
Blackened Cajun Tempeh Bacon	176
Buckwheat Waffles with Gardein Chickenless Strips	177
Vegetarian Strawberry Pancakes with Chocolate Almond Spread	178
Chocolate Almond Spread	181
Vegan, Gluten-Free, Dairy-Free Waffle Base	182
Good Morning Granola (Gluten-Free, Low Sugar, High Protein)	185
Cheesy Tofu Scramble	186

Breads

Whole Wheat Baguette	191
Chocolate Banana Bread	192
Farinata	195
Pizza Dough	196

Shot on location in Washington, DC

Cover photo credit: Sarah Matista

Photo credits: Douglas De la Reza and Beverly Kumari

Food stylist: Beverly Kumari

About the Authors

Chef Bev Kumari attended Indiana University Purdue University, where she studied sociology and journalism. She decided on a career change in her early forties, and began attending Daytona State College, where she studied culinary arts and eventually would pursue a career as a Chef.

Chef Bev has had the honor of preparing meals for former Secretary of State Hillary Clinton, senators, five-star generals and military officiants, federal officers of courts, and other politicians as well as the comptroller of the United States.

She currently works as a sous chef in the Washington, DC, area.

"The plate is the canvass, and the food is the paint. I am an artist, and I paint each dish with the colors of food." (Chef Bev Kumari).

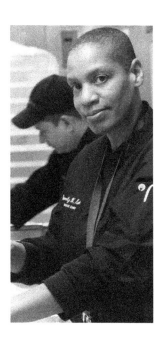

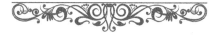

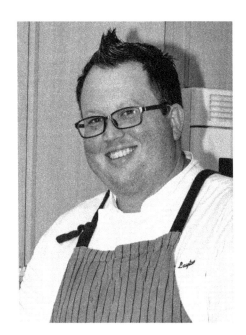

Chef JJ Layton received his formal culinary training at Le Cordon Bleu. However, his love for cuisine began at the age of eight, attached to his mother's apron strings and a loaf of banana bread.

He is continuously amazed at the depth and variety of flavors that Mother Nature has brought to us in the bounty of the garden.

Currently he is the executive chef in Central Florida.

"Good food feeds the body; great food feeds the soul"
(Chef JJ Layton).

Chef Abdellah began cooking at a young age, with his father in the family-owned restaurant in Rabat, Morocco, his native city where he was surrounded by the wonders of fresh local ingredients as well as the aromas of the Moroccan spice markets.

A graduate of the Culinary Institute of America (CIA), where he received two degrees, Chef Abdellah has trained and worked at the Le Cirque, L'espinasse, the late Windows of the World, Mayflower, and St. Regis Hotels, the five-star Mary Elanie at the Phoenician Resorts in Scottsdale, Arizona.

Abdellah is currently the Executive Chef at the largest Marriott Hotel property, the Wardman Park, where he develops recipes showcasing more seasonal meals and some with a hint of his native Moroccan flavors.

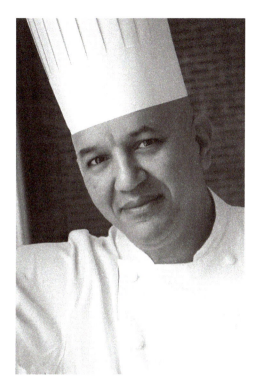

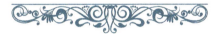

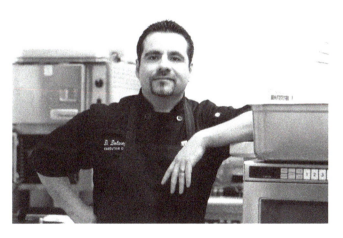

Chef Douglas De la Reza was born in La Paz, Bolivia, where he attended culinary school. At the age of twenty-four, he began working with a Michelin Chef in Washington, DC.

At the age of thirty-two, he began working as an Executive Chef for an exclusive and well-known catering company in the DC area.

Chef Doug looks to the future with enthusiasm, as his retirement plans include building a self-sustaining farm and culinary school in Austin, Texas, utilizing compact containers as the school's foundation.

"Sustainable food is the future of a healthier community" (Chef Douglas De la Reza).

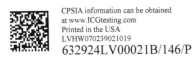

CPSIA information can be obtained
at www.ICGtesting.com
Printed in the USA
LVHW070239021019
632924LV00021B/146/P